FUNCTIONS of a MANAGER in Occupational Therapy

THIRD EDITION

FUNCTIONS of a MANAGER in Occupational Therapy

THIRD EDITION

Edited by

Karen Jacobs, EdD, OTR/L, CPE, FAOTA
Sargent College of Health and Rehabilitation Sciences
Department of Occupational Therapy
Boston University
Boston, Massachusetts

Martha K. Logigian, MS, OTR/L
Department of Occupational Therapy and Physical Therapy
Clinical Associates of the Finger Lakes
Victor, New York

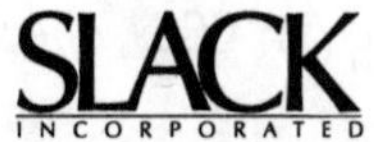

6900 Grove Road, Thorofare, NJ 08086

Publisher: John H. Bond
Editorial Director: Amy E. Drummond
Senior Associate Editor: Jennifer J. Cahill

The work SLACK publishes is peer reviewed. Prior to publication, recognized leaders in the field, educators, and clinicians provide important feedback on the concepts and content that we publish. We welcome feedback on this work.

Functions of a manager in occupational therapy/[edited by] Karen Jacobs, Martha K. Logigian.--3rd ed.
p. cm.
Includes bibliographical references and index.
ISBN 1-55642-374-8
1. Occupational therapy services--Administration. I. Jacobs, Karen. II. Logigian, Martha K.
RM735.6.F86 1999
362.1'78--dc21 99-12759

Printed in the United States of America

Published by: SLACK Incorporated
6900 Grove Road
Thorofare, NJ 08086-9447 USA
Telephone: 856-848-1000
Fax: 856-853-5991
http://www.slackinc.com

Contact SLACK Incorporated for more information about other books in this field or about the availability of our books from distributors outside the United States.

Last digit is print number: 10 9 8 7 6 5 4 3

Dedication

We dedicate this edition to our co-workers
who have made our jobs easier
and help us grow and laugh.

Contents

Acknowledgments

We gratefully acknowledge the contribution of our contributing authors and the support of our publisher, SLACK Incorporated. Specifically, we would like to thank John Bond, Publisher; Amy Drummond, Editorial Director; Jennifer Cahill, Senior Associate Editor; and Debra Christy, Managing Editor for their continued support and assistance. A special thanks to Janice McInnis, Barbara Odaka, Heidi Kaplow, Doris Schannen, and our families for their patience and understanding, and Patricia Wernig for her technical assistance.

Contributing Authors

Gail M. Bloom, MA, OTR/L
Occupational Therapy Consultant
Andover, Massachusetts

Mary Farrell, MS, OTR/L
Notre Dame College
Manchester, New Hampshire

Thomas F. Fisher, MS, OTR/L, CCM, FAOTA
Eastern Kentucky University
Richmond, Kentucky

James F. Gardner, PhD
Council on Quality and Leadership in Support for People with Disabilities
Towson, Maryland

Karen Jacobs, EdD, OTR/L, CPE, FAOTA
Sargent College of Health and Rehabilitation Sciences
Department of Occupational Therapy
Boston University
Boston, Massachusetts

Martha K. Logigian, MS, OTR/L
Department of Occupational Therapy and Physical Therapy
Clinical Associates of the Finger Lakes
Victor, New York

Nancy MacRae, MS, OTR/L, FAOTA
Occupational Therapy Department
University of New England
Biddeford, Maine

Wilma Rizal-Bilton, MS, OTR/L
Rehabilitation Services
Brigham and Women's Hospital
Boston, Massachusetts

Mary Hayes Whinery, MS, OTR/L, CHT
Hand Management
Brigham and Women's Hospital
Boston, Massachusetts

Mary Jane Youngstrom, MS, OTR/L
University of Kansas Medical Center
OT Education
Kansas City, Kansas

Introduction

The 1990s have presented many challenges to the occupational therapy (OT) manager. Among them are the increasing complexity of all aspects of health care, including documentation requirements, information systems, and fiscal accountability. In addition, attempting to control health care costs has forced individual OT managers to face significant changes.

Decreased revenue has led to continual cost reduction through staff consolidation, increased productivity, affiliations, joint ventures, mergers, and acquisitions. The result is that one must do more with less while remaining proactive with organizational change.

To prepare the OT manager for these and other situations, we have attempted to present the knowledge and skills needed today and in the future.

This book is designed to help you lead the change required, yet at the same time, remain cognizant of a commitment to staff development and student education. Thus we begin the book with chapters on change management and leadership. Prepare your practice for change by honestly assessing winners and losers while developing a change-oriented culture within your group. You are the leader setting direction for the staff's work and accountability. With this in mind, the chapter on marketing strategies should be useful, as today your customers are not only your clients, but your purchasers as well. The chapter on cost management will provide a foundation for fiscal analysis—understanding how money is spent will facilitate economy of service.

Do not lose sight of your most valuable resource—an excellent staff. Energize and shape staff with appropriate supervision. Help the staff to decrease duplication of services while articulating what occupational therapists (OTs) do best. Good supervisors are a manager's ally in that they are critical to the recruitment and retention of clinically effective and efficient therapists.

Determine ethical solutions to problems, including those that are related to the demands for cost-effective care. These demands have led to increased pressure for detailed documentation as a means of explaining the need for OT services and to enhance reimbursement.

Managing personnel requires that we hire and retain qualified therapists. Yet at the same time, we must measure, improve, and demonstrate quality care. This is done through the implementation of monitoring programs that evaluate the efficacy of intervention models and staffing patterns (Schell & Slater, 1998). The OT manager must realize that it is not just the client's well-being which must be taken into account, but the interests of the family, employer, third party payer, and community at large.

For the new OT program we have included a chapter on program development. This is particularly important in these times of re-engineering and multisystem management. The final chapter is on student education. We must provide competent fieldwork experience for students because they are the profession's future.

With a good understanding of management functions, we believe that you will be able to extend your performance beyond traditional departmental management and become a leader in your organization, demonstrating the contributions of OT in a variety of service programs. Lead your staff in providing a full-service continuum of care at the highest quality, yet at a reasonable cost. Facilitate their understanding of the need for network building, cross-training, and competency development. Flexibility and responsiveness are key for you as manager and for you to instill among your staff. We hope that with insight gained from this text and practical management experience, you will help lead OT into the next millennium.

References

Schell, B. A., & Slater, D. Y. (1998). Management competencies required of administrative and clinical practitioners in the new millennium. *Am J Occup Ther, 52*(9), 744-750.

CHAPTER 1

Change Management

Martha K. Logigian, MS, OTR/L

Change creates challenges and opportunities. How we manage change will influence the outcome. In other words, we can make things happen or watch them happen and wonder why. Yet, as Machiavelli wrote, "There is nothing more difficult to take in hand, more perilous to conduct, or more uncertain in its success than to take the lead in the introduction of a new order of things" (Dobyns, 1990).

We cannot change the past or that people will act in a certain way. However, we can approach change with a positive attitude. Attitude can make or break an individual, department, or company. In fact, companies that have a positive attitude toward change are considered innovative and most likely to succeed, and innovative companies have best practices in common (Kanter, 1983). They foster change based on a clear focus, open communication, network formation (e.g., teams and cross-training), decentralization of resources, and power sharing. For example, when asked what accounted for the success of corporate restructuring, exemplary companies responded that:

- It was based on a clear business imperative.
- They handled downsizing in a humane manner.
- Senior management was visible.
- There was a clearly articulated vision and objectives.
- Line management was committed to the process.
- There were effective employee communications.
- Employees were involved in the change (*Best Practices in Corporate Restructuring*, 1993).

Today, occupational therapy (OT) managers are confronting the same dramatic changes that have occurred in other industries. We must learn from other businesses that have experienced change and positioned themselves in a winning mode. The key to winning is to face change head-on, not wait for it to be imposed. Aggressive action will fare better than a wait-and-see action. A proactive approach to change enables it to become our ally rather than our adversary.

Health Care Changes

For our purposes, change is defined as planned or unplanned response to pressures or forces. The health care industry is currently undergoing major transformational change similar in scope to the change that occurred in the last decade to the automobile and steel industries. It has brought about a highly competitive marketplace that is driven by price, and is significantly influenced by the major reductions that have taken place in Medicare and Medicaid, with more on the horizon. This has led to institutional restructuring, departmental downsizing, and cost containment. There is a shift from episodic, specialty care to preventive, primary care and inpatient to outpatient care that spans the entire continuum. Although in the past the focus of health care was on a patient care model based on illness, the number of inpatient admissions, and available beds, it is now a model that focuses on wellness, outcomes, and health status.

The paradigm has changed from the old **cost + profit = price** to the new **price - cost = profit**. At the same time there are continually rising market expectations for high-quality, cost-effective patient care. As a result, all areas of health care are being examined for potential savings. This has led to an emphasis to decrease the use of expensive ancillary services as a means of controlling cost. In fact, the question now being asked is, "Do we need these interventions at all?" As managers we must be prepared for these changes and be responsive to them. We need to identify the value of the service we provide from a functional and economic perspective and the cost/benefit of long-term outcomes.

Management Changes

Management paradigms have also changed from a mechanical model following World War II to a biological model moving toward a social model emphasizing interactions. The focus of the last is that people are good and doing their best and want to be a part of the change that occurs. It is management's job to involve the workers in problem solving and facing the future. People change the organization because people are the organization. And people have predictable responses to change that must be taken into account. The overt physical change can be easily defined and measured. However, the psychological adaptation necessary to accept change is often ignored, yet critical to the success of change (Carr, 1994).

The personnel adaptation to change can be divided into three phases, the first being ending (i.e., the familiar ends), and there is a sense of loss due to a break with what has been considered safe or accepted practice. A change requires us to function in unfamiliar ways, which implies taking risks. The second phase is ambiguity. As the old situation begins to change, the individual feels adrift and confused. Late in this stage there is acknowledgment that there has been a loss that brings about grief and opportunity. The final phase is acceptance—a new beginning in which one can renew learning within a new paradigm. Resistance is the most common initial response to change, and organizations are tempted to push workers into acceptance rather than allowing them to work through the phases of change. The lesson for managers is to implement appropriate strategies for dealing with resistance, such as communication with and participation of employees, as well as supportive strategies (Carr, 1989).

Today's successful manager is able to build consensus for a planned change by recognizing the need to form common ground by using different approaches to influence different people. The manager is able to think ideas through from a systems perspective, anticipating obstacles and seeking to persuade vested stakeholders. Understanding the organization and the health care environment can help to manage the internal work environment, while data can be used as the basis for a well-reasoned argument. There needs to be understanding of the formal and informal structures of decision making, and knowledge of how to respond to requests and needs of other caregivers.

Responsibility for leading change must be distributed appropriately to promote participation. In addition, the manager understands different behaviors of employees during time of change and helps them to move from a sense of loss, danger, and fear to opportunity, exploration, and commitment to a new beginning (*BWH Compass*, 1996).

For example, if we use the best practice model noted earlier, we need to first clearly identify the imperative forcing the change, such as loss of revenue due to Medicare cuts. A clear business imperative makes communicating difficult messages easier and facilitates employee buy-in to solutions (*Best Practices in Corporate Restructuring*, 1993). Second, any changes should be handled humanely (i.e., no across-the-board cuts, but rather thoughtful continual renewal). This can be done by establishing a team to make recommendations to meet the challenge. The purpose of the team is to group think systems changes which are necessary steps to successful transition to a reorganized system (Johnstone, Rosen, & DeFelippo, 1992). This team should be led by the person in charge so that senior management is visible. The vision and objectives for the change must be clearly delineated. This may reflect the organization as a whole (i.e., "The entire organization is losing money, what can we do about it? What is our vision for the future and what are the objectives that can be identified to get us to this vision?").

Members of the team should include persons who are affected by the change and who can foster ownership of the change. They should have an investment in the change outcome and work hard to make their results successful. Participation on the team can help allay fears resulting from the uncertainty of the change taking place. A well-chosen team provides a pool of knowledge which may include overlooked perspectives (Johnstone et al., 1992).

Line management is involved through participation on the team or for organization-wide issues on subgroups. The use of a team also provides management with an opportunity to enhance employees' understanding of the organization's goals and external forces that impact those goals. They meet with employees individually and in small groups to hear their ideas and concerns. At this time, information can be disseminated about the impending change. Effective communication takes place by sharing each step of the process with all employees on a regular and ongoing basis. There should be a flow of information from team members to peers and vice versa. Teams should meet regularly and have an agenda, which includes time for new issues and invited experts to speak. Quality, frequency, and timeliness of communications are critical, particularly during a period of great change. It is management's job to involve workers in solving problems and facing the future.

Strategic Thinking

There is a tendency to overestimate immediate change and underestimate the effect of long-term change. Ensure that steps taken provide for fundamental, not cosmetic, change (*Best Practices in Corporate Restructuring*, 1993). As such, strategic thinking is particularly useful in managing change. Among the strategies to consider are:

- Direct the movement of change, do not fight it.
- Develop an intuitive sense of timing to know when to cut through ambiguity.
- Develop a long-range approach considering advantages/disadvantages of actions.
- Become a master of leverage using measured force at critical moments toward the desired goal.
- Try to influence others rather than control them.
- Stay in control and do not let frustrations, fears, or image prompt emotional reactions.
- Be action oriented by trying to solve a problem, learning from the outcome (Fine, 1988).

To utilize strategic planning in change management, a critical feature is systematic thinking and commitment of resources to actions. Become a systems thinker. Articulate and encourage a common perspective where individuals see themselves as part of a system and build upon each other's efforts. Actively seek information, and logically plan and organize work. Recognize the interconnections of activities. Utilize quantitative data and creative problem solving and planning methods which stretch beyond the familiar and safe (Fine, 1988).

Avoid mental blinders such as "my reality is the reality" and separating self from external reality. Move away from focusing on events rather than process (i.e., what vs. why) as well as fragmentation thinking (i.e., group vs. individual). It is of no help to believe that the enemy is out there or big change requires big action. Do not indulge in the illusion of control or spend undue time worrying or speculating about possibilities. Instead, focus on the future and the goals for improving care and services while managing costs (Orlikoff, 1996).

Learning Centers

Figure 1-1 presents management learning centers (*BWH Compass*, 1996). It is based on managerial competencies required for successful leadership to support an institution's strategic vision. This is a model that some organizations have found useful to incorporate as part of their management strategy to deal with change. Such a system is based on competencies that allow the learning necessary to drive business improvement. The scope of managing change includes the definition and development of a way of managing that capitalizes on change as a positive force, encouraging and building upon resilience.

Performance indicators highlight important competencies for an individual manager. Each center of learning interrelates with the others in the same way that cooperative work groups function in industry. Change management requires that the manager communicate effectively, consider the impact of actions taken, drive action, and use data persuasively.

The most important trait among excellent companies is an action orientation (Peters & Waterman, 1982). It is useful to develop an action plan to deal with change. Planning throughout the change process should have a broad perspective. Identifying and labeling foreseeable problems early in the planning process reduces the tendency to solve problems impulsively. Change can become incremental and disjointed if it is not incorporated as part of the strategy and planning (Johnstone et al., 1992). When a plan is developed to deal with the situation demanding change, communication within the workforce is essential. This is two-way communication so that all employees feel a part of the process. In addition to verbal exchange, written minutes of meetings should be posted so that all can be appraised of the situation. Thus, keeping the competencies from Figure 1-1 in mind, an action plan for the current health care environment includes the following:

- Analyze the situation.
- Develop a shared vision.
- Convey urgency.
- Identify and support strong leadership.
- Line up a network of sponsorship.
- Formulate a detailed implementation plan.
- Reinforce change (*BWH Compass*, 1996; Kotter, 1995).

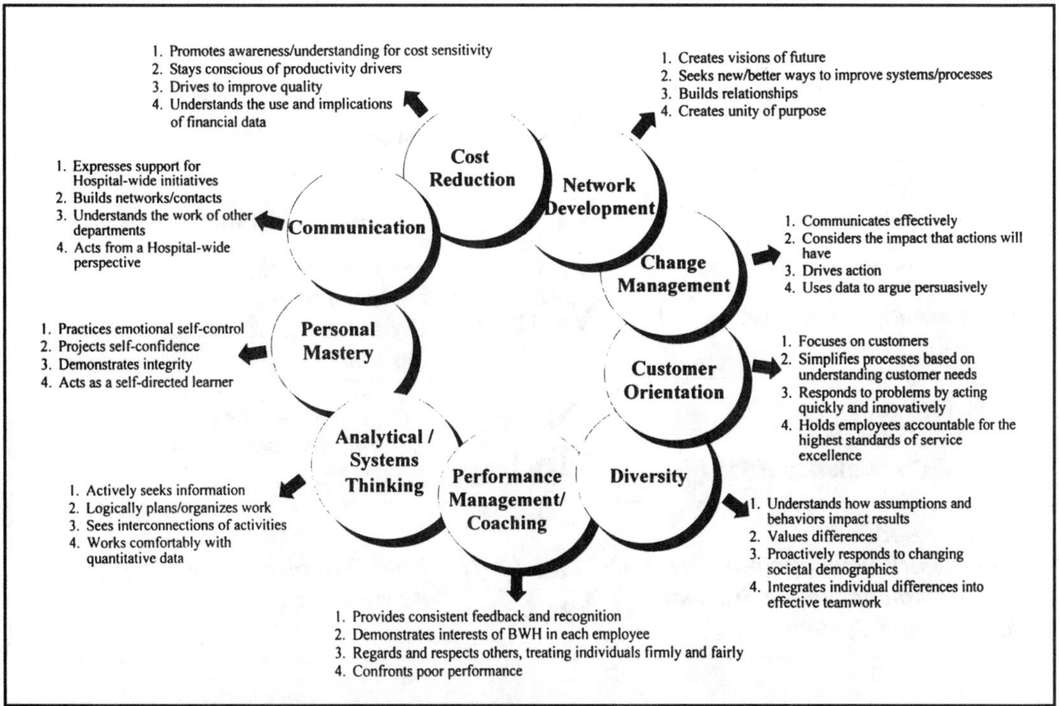

Figure 1-1. Learning centers: Performance indicators for competencies. Courtesy of Brigham and Women's Hospital, Boston, MA.

When there is a systematic agenda for change within an organization, there is a mission that defines organizational goals and objectives. There is a vision that defines leadership focus. There are values or operating principles that demonstrate the underlying beliefs and drive the organization to its missions and vision. There is a model for how the organization will think, look, and act. Figures 1-2a and 1-2b, for example, are designed to be a generative model that is organic, continuous from patient to employee, and competency based. Finally, there are strategies/tactics which identify how the organization will achieve its mission, such as by using a learning system model.

Corporate Renewal

Static changes as are implied by the word "restructuring," suggest one-time, lasting events. When people see change as an event rather than a process, their behavior is often reactive and shaped to accommodate the particular event, such as the integration of two work functions or a new boss. This can set up potentially false expectations that soon everything will be okay. This conceptual framework for organizational change requires employees to adapt passively to change.

On the other hand, when people see change as a process, the behaviors are less reactive and more proactive. The latter include activities such as problem solving, experimentation, after the fact discussions on successes and failures, knowledge and technology transfer, and the integration of identified best practices. In other words, structural change can be more successful within the context of the process of becoming an excellent company, department, or unit. This process is what is known as corporate renewal.

Corporate renewal is an analogy to that which occurs in nature. Surviving this circle of life is the challenge to corporate life. It involves continually redefining one's understanding of the com-

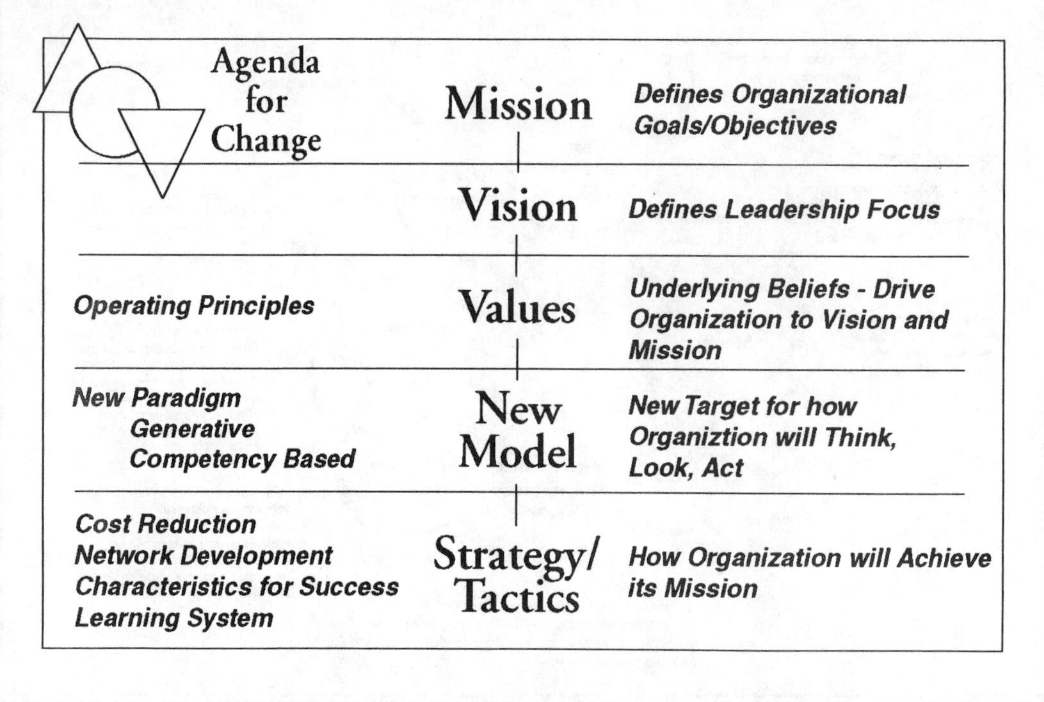

Figure 1-2a. Agenda for change. Courtesy of Brigham and Women's Hospital, Boston, MA.

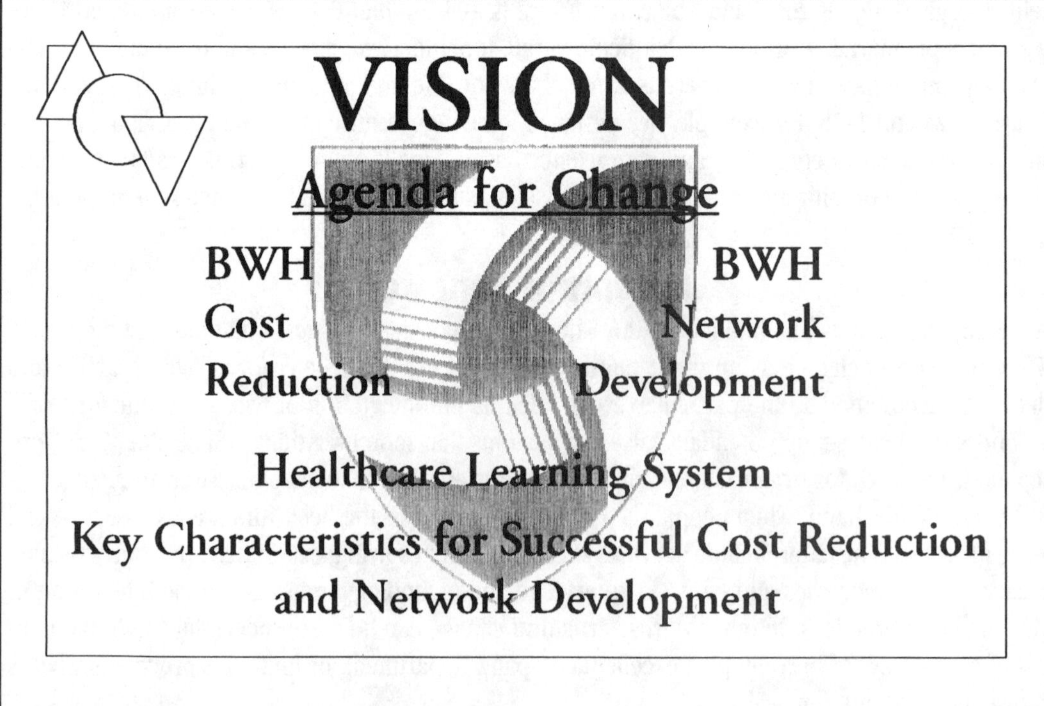

Figure 1-2b. Agenda for change. Courtesy of Brigham and Women's Hospital, Boston, MA.

pany's key constituencies and their needs, as well as what value the organization delivers to meet those needs. One must continually ask how that value can be enhanced and what activities detract from providing value to those constituencies. Decisions that evolve from these questions may be harsh in their impact on people and are not meant to be a quick fix or one-time event. Rather it is a process of continual organizational change that can be harnessed if people learn how to engage in and embrace renewal behaviors. Learning must occur as motivation is not enough. One must be able to participate fully through knowledge of the process. Thus, a learning organization fosters an environment conducive to learning by providing time for learning and skills with which to learn. Organizational boundaries must be opened through cross-organizational teams and conferences, including suppliers and customers. Programs should be initiated with explicit learning goals. Finally, rewards and recognition should be adjusted to support the value and accomplishment of learning.

Although corporate renewal is designed for the average company, the principles of it can be applied to any size unit. The issue is to invest in developing a learning organization so that no matter what change is encountered, it can survive and be healthy in the future.

Questions

1. Best companies foster change based on:
   a. Open communication
   b. Power sharing
   c. A clear focus
   d. All of the above

2. Change is:
   a. A reaction to a new situation
   b. A planned or unplanned response to pressures
   c. None of the above

3. Change in health care has been brought on by:
   a. Escalating costs
   b. Competitive marketplace
   c. Both a and b
   d. None of the above

4. The current management style is:
   a. Biological model
   b. Mechanical model
   c. Social model

5. The manager today tries to:
   a. Keep employees under control
   b. Build consensus for change
   c. Use disciplinary action to force change
   d. None of the above

6. For organization-wide issues, team participants should include:
   a. Only senior management
   b. Line management
   c. Only employees
   d. Outside consultants

7. A strategy to consider when facing change is:
   a. Develop a long-range approach
   b. Develop a sit back and wait attitude
   c. Force others to think as you do

8. A necessary component of a change situation is:
   a. Learning to help business improvement
   b. Doing nothing
   c. Finding another job

9. An action plan should include:
   a. Analysis of the situation
   b. A shared vision
   c. An implementation plan
   d. All of the above

10. Static change implies:
    a. Constant change
    b. A one-time event
    c. None of the above

Case Study 1

You have just been hired as director of a five-person OT department. Communication is largely gossip and there is little accurate information from the organization's leaders reaching your staff. What should you do about this situation?

Case Study 2

You have been asked to be the supervisor of the OT hand practice which will be moving off-site from the primary practice area. There will be doctors and physical therapists (PTs) in the off-site practice as well. How would you ensure the success of this move?

References

Best practices in corporate restructuring. (1993). Washington, DC: The Wyatt Co.

BWH compass: A managing tool for implementing change. (1996). Boston: Change Management Learning Center of Brigham and Women's Hospital.

Carr, C. (1989, January). Following through on change. *Training*, 39-42.

Carr, C. (1994, February). Seven keys to successful change. *Training*, 55-60.

Dobyns, L. (1990, June). Ed Deming wants big changes, and he wants them fast. *Smithsonian*, 74-82.

Fine, S. B. (1988). Working the system: A perspective for managing change. *Am J Occup Ther, 42*(7), 417-419.

Johnstone K., Rosen H., & DeFelippo, A. (1992). Management of change in a large PT department. *Clinical Management, 5*(4), 10-13.

Kanter, R. M. (1983). *The change masters: How people and companies succeed through innovation in the new corporate era*. New York: Simon and Schuster.

Kotter, J. P. (1995, March-April). Why transformation efforts fail. *Harvard Business Review,* 59-67.

Orlikoff, J. E. (1996). *Trends in healthcare*. Orlando, FL: American College of Rheumatology.

Peters, T. J., & Waterman, R. H., Jr. (1982). *In search of excellence*. New York: Harper and Row.

Answer Key

1. d
2. b
3. c
4. c
5. b
6. b
7. a
8. a
9. d
10. b

CHAPTER 2

Leadership and Organizational Behavior

James F. Gardner, PhD

Introduction

The purpose of this chapter is to provide an overview of recent themes in leadership in organizational settings and to relate leadership to organizational behavior. Rather than exploring the detailed research in specific issues or repeating the advice of leading consultants, this chapter will describe an emerging orientation to leadership.

Recent social and economic changes have increased the importance of leadership. In the industrial era with centralized bureaucracies, recognized leaders were at the top of organizational hierarchies. In the post-industrial or knowledge-based society, leadership is distributed throughout organizations.

Computerization has changed the unskilled laborer of mid-century into the knowledge worker of the future. Liberated from physical labor, employees now design better machines and implement new processes that enhance efficiency and effectiveness. Paradoxically, greater technology and automation require greater interpersonal and leadership skills because knowledge workers are freed from the drudgery of the machine to work together, plan, and create new methods for accomplishing the work of the organization.

The Art of Leadership

The contemporary metaphor for leadership is that of art. Vail (1989) uses the performing arts to express the dynamism, fluidity, extraordinary complexity, and fundamental personalness of all organizational change. DePree (1989) notes that leadership is an art, something to be learned over time, not simply by reading books. It is more tribal than science, more a weaving of relationships than an amassing of information. These themes of dynamism, complexity, personalness, and relationships extend throughout much of the leadership literature. They interconnect with other themes of organizational learning, personal reflection, and reframing.

The metaphor of leadership as art indicates that leadership develops through performance and reflection upon performance. Feedback from all representatives in the organization contributes to this reflection and encourages additional leadership development. The metaphor of leadership as an art indicates there are no proven methods of leadership that can address all situations. Like jazz music or improvisational theater, leadership is learned and expanded through the performance itself. Leadership arises not out of textbooks, but rather out of doing and learning from doing.

Leadership and the New Science

The distinction between art and science has traditionally rested on the presence of guidelines and rules that guide decision making. Art is depicted as "figuring it out as you go along" because there are few established guidelines. Science, in contrast, implies a full set of guidelines and empirical evidence to guide choice making. But, the new science of quantum mechanics suggests that science often presents unknowns and that science is more similar to art than dissimilar.

Some portion of contemporary leadership theory is drawn from the transformation in scientific thinking from a world of Newtonian physics to the current world of quantum mechanics and chaos theory. The machine was the metaphor for the Newtonian world. Made up of many smaller parts, the machine could be broken down and analyzed. After examining the individual parts, the machine could be reassembled. Understanding and knowledge followed the analysis of smaller and smaller pieces of reality. This same model was applied to large hierarchical and bureaucratic organizations. Through the use of technical analysis, managers focused understanding on individual functions and units of activity. At the turn of the 20th century, the language of bureaucracy developed which included division of labor, hierarchy of authority, hiring by technical qualifications, and rules and controls. Several years later, Henry Fayol defined the 14 principles of management (Wren, 1979):

1. Division of work
2. Unity of command
3. Remuneration
4. Order
5. Initiative
6. Authority
7. Unity of direction
8. Centralization
9. Equity
10. Esprit de corps
11. Discipline
12. Subordination of individual interest
13. Line of authority
14. Stability of tenure of personnel

The Newtonian world of science and the scientific and administrative theories that supported the bureaucratic world began to falter even as they arose. In the world of quantum theory and chaos theory, the classical notion of ever smaller solid objects dissolves into wave-like patterns of probability. The result is that the sub-atomic particles cannot be understood as isolated entities but must be defined through their relationships (Capra, 1982). The sub-atomic world now appears as a web of relationships within a unified whole (Capra, 1991). Referring to the world of quantum physics, it is noted that connections and relationships rather than separate entities are the fundamental realities of life. Thus, if the physics of our universe is revealing the primacy of relationships, is it any wonder that we are beginning to reconfigure our ideas about management in relational terms. Look carefully at how a workplace organizes its relationships—not its tasks, functions, and hierarchies—one can see the patterns of relationships and the capacities available to form them (Wheatley, 1994).

Leaders are responsible for encouraging the messy and sometimes confusing development of systems of associations and connections within organizations. These systems of interactions cannot be determined ahead of time—they cannot be predicted. In contrast, leaders provide positive energy that enables employees to explore associations and connections. They create an environment where people can learn, take chances, and make mistakes. In this manner people create the relationship systems for accomplishing the work of the organization (Wheatley & Kellner-Rogers, 1996). Leaders are defined as designers, stewards, and teachers, responsible for building organizations where people continually expand their capabilities to understand complexity, clarify vision, and improve shared mental models. They are responsible for learning (Senge, 1990).

This view of leadership is not consistent with the traditional view of leaders as heroic individuals who have answers, make key decisions, energize people, and, ultimately, save the day. This traditional view was based on the belief that the leaders at the top of the hierarchy alone possessed the ability to take command, and the majority of employees at the bottom of the hierarchy were unmotivated and unwilling to take responsibility. Change came from the few great leaders located in the upper echelons of the organization.

Leadership Myths and Competencies

The current genre of management and leadership books and manuals provides a wide range of both sound and dubious advice on how to manage and how to be a leader. Myths are important to note because they are seldom challenged. Competencies are equally important because they are the basics of any "how to" approach to leadership. A number of leadership myths have been identified (McLean & Weitzel, 1991). Some of them are as follows:

- **Charisma is a necessary leadership quality.** Commitment to, and communication of, the organizational vision, and an ability to support and sustain others in quest of the vision, is the more important quality. Vice President Al Gore and Frank Perdue are not particularly charismatic, but they are leaders with visions.
- **Leaders can never be wrong.** Thomas Edison tried more than 3,000 laboratory experiments before he finally produced a working light.
- **Leadership means being consistent.** In a constantly changing world, consistency for consistency sake alone is an organizational anchor. Employees need to know what is expected of them. They need a context for leadership demands. They need to know the vision of the leader.
- **Leaders should always know the goal in advance.** Leaders need visions that give energy to organizations. They need to communicate those visions and build coalitions of support for the organizing visions. However, leaders formulate goals and strategies out of a dialogue with employees, customers, suppliers, and others. Again, our "learning from acting" model indicates that the answers begin to emerge only after the organization begins to act.

Bennis (1989b, 1993) has written frequently on the four competencies of leadership. In a study of 90 effective leaders, Bennis found the following four competencies:

- **The management of attention.** Leaders communicate a focus of commitment that draws people into a consensus. They set forth an unambiguous vision, goal, or direction.

- **The management of meaning.** Leaders communicate that vision through the assembly of facts, concepts, and anecdotes into meaning for followers. Leaders use metaphors, stories, models, and symbols to clarify visions. They make visions tangible and real to others.
- **The management of trust.** Leaders must display consistency in their values and vision. This reliability over time infuses trust into the organization. Trust is an essential part of all organizations.
- **The management of self.** Self-awareness and self-dialogue are critical. Knowledge of one's own skills, attitudes, limitations, and lack of understanding is the basis for learning. Knowing when and how to act provides the beginning of learning.

From Warrior to Philosopher

In contrast to the image of leader as warrior, current depictions cast the leader as knowledgeable philosopher. Leadership is described in terms of self-knowledge and reflection. Potential leaders are urged to develop a personal mission statement. This personal mission statement defines the values and principles that guide the leader in day-to-day decision making. Possession of these core values and principles enables the leader to move quickly and decisively in rapidly changing environments. The key to the ability to change is a changeless sense of who you are, what you are about, and what you value (Covey, 1990).

The leader as philosopher builds upon, and perhaps modifies, these core values by engaging in continuous learning about oneself. Leadership is described in terms of self-knowledge and self-discovery. It is a process of inventing oneself through self-knowledge (Bennis, 1989b). The search for leadership in oneself is a quest for self-development (Kouzes & Posner, 1987). Self-reflection leads the individual to the possibilities for change(Wheatley & Kellner-Rogers, 1996). The ability of such people to be natural leaders is the by-product of a lifetime of effort, effort to develop conceptual and communication skills, reflect on personal values, and align personal behavior with values (Senge, 1990).

Self-discovery and personal awareness is a continuous process of questioning basic assumptions. At times, it is similar to dialogue with oneself. Leaders routinely ask such questions as:

- What are my strengths and weaknesses?
- How committed am I to my basic values and mission? To those of the organization?
- How much do I really understand about this organization? The external environment?
- Am I prepared to handle the complex problems facing the organization?
- Am I the person to lead at this time (Kouzes & Posner, 1987)?

Other questions are more for a self-dialogue:

- What do you believe are the qualities of leadership?
- What were the turning points in your life?
- What role has failure played in your life?
- How did you learn (Bennis, 1989b)?

The leader as philosopher approaches mistakes in a manner altogether differently than the leader as warrior. The leader as warrior fears mistakes because they threaten the leader's claim to invincibility. In reality, mistakes and leadership are not mutually exclusive. But, when they become mutually exclusive, leaders and top managers avoid mistakes by not acting. Not acting precludes any further learning and erodes the process of self-discovery. The path to learning and self-discovery requires decision making and action, and these, in turn, require permission to make mistakes while engaging in the journey. Knowledge is nothing without action. Nothing changes until you do something. What you do will directly determine what you learn (Belasco & Stayer, 1993).

The philosopher leader does not worry about mistakes because leaders put all of their energy into their task (Bennis, 1989b). Leaders stay focused on the positive goals. They avoid wasting negative energy on worry and mistakes. In addition, leaders treat mistakes as opportunities for learning. Successful managers reframe mistakes as the opportunity for self-discovery through decision making and action. Leaders do not seek failures, but they recognize the opportunity to learn from each failure. Belasco and Stayer (1993) recall establishing a "Shot in the Foot Award" for the employee who both made the biggest mistake and learned the most from that mistake. In analyzing the leadership style of Moses, it is noted that his pattern of leadership was not a matter of going from one success to another but of salvaging some success from each defeat (Wildavsky, 1984).

Moses endured defeat after defeat because of his vision or purpose. The vision is a target that beckons (Bennis & Nanus, 1985). The vision is different than the personal values or principles. The vision is the definition of where the organization belongs. The role of the leader is to guarantee the vision of the organization. At times, this will require charm and charisma. At other times, leaders may need to be hard and insensitive to keep the company consistent with the vision and goals (Deal & Kennedy, 1982). Leadership style may change with the circumstances, but it always serves the mission and goals of the organization.

The role of the leader is to develop a shared vision and goal for the organization. Leaders need buy-in from members of the organization around the vision and goals. Clear visions and futuristic goals are pointless if they are not communicated, understood, and shared. This indicates the distinction between visionaries and leaders. Visionaries develop futuristic goals and visions, but they stop short of communication and building coalitions around the visions. Leaders communicate and develop coalitions of support around energizing visions. Without the shared vision, employees will go about incorporating their own interpretation of the vision into the fabric of the organization. Multiple definitions of vision dissipate organizational energy into different, and sometimes contradictory, directions.

The importance of vision points to the difference between management and leadership. Management without leadership is like straightening deck chairs on the Titanic (Covey, 1990). Management is doing the job right. It is a matter of technique, method, analysis, and review. Leadership, in contrast, is doing the right job. Leadership requires vision and values, synthesis, and feedback. The difference between leaders and managers is demonstrated by describing a group of workers cutting and hacking their way through a jungle. As producers and problem solvers, they cut through the obstacles to accomplish their job. The managers do the planning, sharpen the tools, train in brush hacking, and establish work and compensation schedules. But the leader is the one who climbs the tallest tree, surveys the entire situation, and yells "Wrong jungle" (Bennis, 1989a, 1989b; Drucker, 1954).

Good management cannot create leaders. Instead, good management can create environments in which leaders and leadership qualities can incubate and evolve. Because leaders are made by their experience, their learning in action, organizations need to provide potential leaders with the opportunities to learn through experience in an environment that permits growth and change (Bennis, 1989a).

Organizational Behavior

Organizational behavior refers to the interactions of individuals and groups in organizations. The leaders' understanding of organizational behavior is important because the workplace is changing very rapidly. Successful leaders will understand the change and transformation of the future and mold their leadership style around the culture of the new workplace. Social changes in the emerging workplace culture is occurring at a great pace. Call it re-engineering, restructuring, transformation flattening, downsizing, rightsizing, a quest for global competitiveness—it is real, radical, and arriving every day at a company near you (Huey, 1993).

The workplace is changing so rapidly because of new technology, more diversity, and greater customer demand. Computers and information technology are replacing hierarchical bureaucracies with extended information networks. In some instances, the borders between companies disappear in the electronic wirescape. In addition, increased women in the workforce, increased immigration, and changing social norms are creating greater cultural, sexual, and racial diversity in the workplace. Finally, the new customer demand for quality means that companies must now satisfy customers in terms of quality, service, and cost.

Organizational Behavior and Individuals

Individual workers have basic attributes of motivation, aptitude, personality, values, attitudes, and perceptions. While the attributes are all important, leaders pay particular attention to values and perceptions. Values are the global beliefs that guide action and judgment in different situations. Perception is the process through which people input, process, and analyze information. Values provide the beginning of the perceptual process and contribute to the schemas that people use to sort information. Schemas are like computer software which arrange information in various patterns. Values and schemas guide our perceptual process.

Successful leaders recognize that organizations consist of people with different values, schemas, and perceptions. When confronted with a solid, objective reality, different people perceive the reality differently. In addition, successful leaders understand their own values, schemas, and perceptual biases through self-reflection and learning from both successes and failures.

Organizational Behavior and Groups

Understanding individuals and developing effective interpersonal skills increase leader effectiveness. However, for successful managers and leaders, the focus for action is the group rather than the individual. Understanding group behavior requires attention to the stages of group development and group norms. There are four stages of group development:

1. **Forming stage.** Leaders are challenged in managing the initial entry of different individuals into the new group.
2. **Storming stage.** Leaders are challenged to manage the high emotions and tension of group members as they each search for status and role.
3. **Initial integration stage.** Leaders are challenged by relationships and tasks as norms for behavior are established.
4. **Total integration.** With norms set, leaders are challenged to move the group to continuously learn, reflect, and improve.

Successful leaders understand that groups evolve through this sequence. Leaders can cope with multiple teams at different levels of development. Sometimes leaders take teams back to the beginning if there has been significant change in membership. In addition, the storming in phase two of the development is a natural occurrence. The interpersonal difficulties and the questioning of authority are often difficult, but they are part of the natural process of group development. The leadership role in these stages of group development is to explain the evolutionary nature of the process, guide the group through its current phase, and steer a middle road through either suppression of conflict or abandonment of the group to its own self-destruction.

Most individuals belong to various groups, and the groups' behaviors are governed by unwritten rules, known as norms. Group norms guide individual behavior and action. Individuals adopt these norms when they decide to join the group. Conscious and unconscious peer pressure maintain the group norms.

Norms exist outside the formal set of organizational policy and procedure. Group norms cannot be changed by issuing new policy and procedure or by ordinary supervisory methods. This explains the phenomenon of the futility of attempting to change group behavior by sending representatives to workshops and seminars. Members return full of knowledge and enthusiasm, but then they hit the hard wall of organizational norms, and the excitement and innovation vanish.

Leaders change group norms by creating opportunities for groups to engage in a collective re-examination of their own performance, and by identifying alternative norms that might better meet the group's needs. The leader cannot impose his or her norms on the group. In contrast, the leader enables the group to meet and develop its own new norms. The following points can guide the renorming process:

- All participants governed by the norms actively participate in the renorming process.
- Leaders and managers responsible for final actions participate.
- Participants involved in the process must be affected by the norms.
- Objective information is most valuable.
- Opportunity to express anger and frustration as natural by-products is offered.
- Agreements on new norms are explicit.
- Changes are monitored and measured.

Reframing Organizational Behavior

There is a three-step process for making basic changes in groups and organizations. The first stage is unfreezing, preparing the organization for change. The leader disconfirms existing values, perceptions, or norms. This unfreezing is facilitated by organizational crisis, environmental pressure, or a competitor's innovation and can occur over time. Leaders can also promote the unfreezing by gathering people together and re-examining organizational norms through the process previously discussed. In the second stage of the process, leaders introduce an alternative to the existing values, perceptions, and norms. This changing stage depends upon the success of the previous unfreezing stage. Without successful unfreezing, the change stage will be plagued with resistance and hostility. The final stage is one of refreezing as the new values, perceptions, and norms are frozen in place. Evaluation and monitoring systems that report success to the group reinforce performance. The refreezing process can be prolonged. Incomplete refreezing can result in backsliding to former values, perceptions, and norms (Lewin, 1951).

The prerequisite for successful organizational change is the ability of the leader to mentally reframe organizational situations. This mental reframing proceeds the organizational change; it enables the leader to see multiple values, perceptions, and norms operating at the same time within the organization. Reframing provides the leader with multiple opportunities and courses for action. Behind every effort to improve organizations lies a set of assumptions or theories about how organizations work and what might make work better (Bolman & Deal, 1991).

The term theory is similar to the previous term, schemas. Theories are the organizing models that explain why organizations work and behave the way they do. Like software, our theories and schemas align data and information in certain patterns. Four prevailing organizational schemas have been identified:

1. A **structural** orientation emphasizes goals, roles, technology, and organizational structure. Organizations exist to achieve goals. Organizational structure is determined by a mix of goals, technology, and environment. Organizational behavior is rational. Planning and analysis lead to goal formation.
2. A **human resource** approach emphasizes the interdependence between organizations and people. The management focuses on developing a better fit between people's personal attributes and the work roles and responsibilities.
3. A **political** perspective views organization life as a contest over allocation of scarce resources. Organizations are coalitions of groups and individuals. Goal formation is determined by the dominant political coalition.
4. A **symbolic** approach focuses on the meaning of events rather than on the event itself. Attempts to create organization cohesion through structure, power, or human relations are limited (Bolman & Deal, 1991).

These four frames provide different approaches to the basic organizational requirements of organizational management, group interactions, and conflict resolutions. Consider the following responses to basic managerial issues of management of organizations, group interactions, and conflict present in Table 2-1.

These schemas provide templates or software that give order to the many experiences of our work life. Different employees will use these different schemas to interpret and explain the same information or events. Consider, for example, an OT department within a rehabilitation hospital that has recently joined an alliance of long-term care and rehabilitation hospitals. New management, new financial management, and possible personnel changes are rumored. Some managers interpret these events in a structural frame and propose that structure be examined and streamlined. They propose new job descriptions and reporting relationships. In contrast, those influenced by the human relations perspective will argue that new management meet with all the employees, explain the new structure, and listen to the therapists' concerns about the new organization. Some will propose a task force to monitor morale. Those attracted to the political frame will attempt to forge coalitions to preserve and extend power and influence. Finally, those working in a symbolic frame will attempt to explain the meaning of the change and use symbols or visions of the future to rally support.

This ability to reframe extends beyond organizational and management applications. The ability to reframe and look at reality from different perspectives has significant clinical applications. The occupational therapist's (OT's) leadership capability is enhanced when clinical practice can be examined from multiple perspectives. A four-frame analysis of disability enables us to understand the diversity within the health and human services community on issues related to disability (Daniels, 1991). The four different interpretations of disability are found in Table 2-2.

Table 2-1
Organizational Behavior Associated with Different Frames

Management of Organizations	
Structural	Manage through rules
Human Resource	Manage through group norms
Political	Manage through power
Symbolic	Manage through symbols
Group Interactions	
Structural	Stress order through structure
Human Resource	Stress harmony through personal interaction
Political	Stress coalition building
Symbolic	Lead through use of symbols
Conflict	
Structural	Reduce through restructuring and rules
Human Resource	Reduce through interpersonal interventions
Political	Use conflict to build coalitions
Symbolic	Reduce through development of supraordinate goals

Table 2-2
Disability Frames

The Individual Defect Paradigm	
Focus	The individual with the disability
Problem	Inability to perform major life activities such as walking, working, learning
Solution	Restoration of function and adaptation to disability
Strategies	Specialized treatment for people with disabilities
Outcome	Improved function
Key Players	Professionals and specialists
Key Words	Functional limitation, vocational evaluation, acceptance, and adjustment
The Community/Social Unit Paradigm	
Focus	The family, community, and service system decision makers
Problem	Disruption of natural relationships through highly specialized services in highly specialized places
Solution	Community inclusion, family-centered and driven supports
Strategies	Self-advocacy, community involvement
Outcome	Community ownership of problems and solutions
Key Players	People with disabilities, family, friends, ordinary citizens
Key Words	Inclusion, self-advocacy, natural supports
The Technology/Ecology Paradigm	
Focus	Systems of information, financing, implementation of assistive technology
Problem	Failure of the service delivery system to provide access to assistive technology
Solution	Access to tools and technology that promote economic, social, community goals
Strategies	Integrated service delivery systems responsive to people with disabilities
Outcome	More individual choice and control
Key Players	Technology specialists, instructors, people with disabilities
Key Words	Consumer driven, adaptive, computer
The Individual Rights Paradigm	
Focus	The society, laws, systems, and relationships
Problem	Persistent and pervasive discrimination against people with disabilities
Solution	Access to economic, social, and educational opportunity
Strategies	Civil rights legislation, litigation, policy reform, consciousness raising, political action
Outcome	Full rights and responsibilities of citizenship
Key Players	Advocates, lawyers, community organizers
Key Words	Equity and opportunity, rights and remedies, discrimination, due process

None of these four schemas related to management or disability are better than another. Each provides a different interpretation of events, and each suggests a different response. Understanding the four frames and understanding how others think in the different frames extends leadership capability. When managers learn how to see other points of view, they increase effectiveness. When managers can reframe situations and analyze situations from different frames, they can generate multiple responses to situations.

Conclusion

The ability to reframe and understand other perspectives rests on self-awareness and internal reflection. Until managers understand their own biases and tendencies to think in only narrow frames, they cannot begin the process of reframing. Thus leadership and reframing rest on the same processes of self-discovery. The reflection of leadership and reframing provides greater opportunities for analysis and explanation. This enables leaders to understand and value other points of view. In fact, leaders can reframe oppositional behavior as thinking in a different frame than one's own. Finally, the ability to reframe provides the leader with multiple strategies and solutions for problems and challenges in organizations.

Questions

1. Which term best characterizes leadership?
   a. Boldness
   b. Science
   c. Art
   d. Contingency theory

2. Leadership is learned through:
   a. Leadership seminars
   b. Performance itself
   c. Academic journals
   d. Mentors

3. The new science suggests that leadership is a study in:
   a. Individual performance
   b. Quantitative methods
   c. Relationships
   d. Leadership traits

4. In the emerging post-industrial, knowledge-based society, leadership is:
   a. Located throughout the organization
   b. Located at the mid-level management position
   c. Located at the top and bottom of the organization
   d. Located in the management information division

5. Which of the following is true?
   a. Charisma is a necessary leadership quality
   b. Leaders can never be wrong
   c. Leaders always know the goals in advance
   d. Strategic planning does not belong with the planning department

6. The leader as philosopher emphasizes:
    a. Both Eastern and Western philosophy
    b. Self-reflection
    c. Learning through acting
    d. Both b and c

7. Schemas are similar to:
    a. Short story plots
    b. Computer software
    c. Leadership strategies
    d. None of the above

8. Organizational norms are:
    a. Unwritten rules for group behavior
    b. Formal organizational rules
    c. Guidelines for leadership behavior
    d. Similar across groups in a company

9. Reframing is a useful skill for leaders because:
    a. It provides insight into the behavior of others
    b. It provides multiple opportunities for action
    c. Both a and b
    d. Neither a nor b

10. Reframing is based on the idea that:
    a. There is a best frame
    b. All frames are equal
    c. People tend to select the frame that best explains the situation or event to them
    d. Certain frames always fit certain situations

Case Study 1—Personal Self-Reflection

As an undergraduate, you have the opportunity to define a process for your own self-reflection and learning as you begin the process of merging work experience with academic preparation. Work experience and professional training are an iterative process. They influence each other. Learning and work go together. Actual experience, self-reflection, and theory and concepts from lifelong learning intermingle.

Previous Leadership Experiences

What opportunities have you had to exercise leadership in the past? What did you learn from those experiences? Thinking back, how could you have reframed mistakes and failures as opportunities to learn and try out new ideas?

Role Models

Are there people in your experience who have served as role models in terms of their leadership? Why do you consider them role models?

Next Steps

Knowing who you are, what are your next steps to learning about yourself in leadership positions? What kind of risk for success or failure can you now tolerate? What is your biggest aversion to failure? How can you reframe your aversion to failure? What do you learn from your successes? How can you learn more in the future?

Lifelong Learning

Leadership requires lifelong learning—about yourself and the world around you. What kind of commitment can you make to lifelong learning? What opportunities can you create for yourself? What aspects of your work and leadership are you most curious about? What about your personal life?

Learning Through Acting

Academic preparation for your career stresses proficiency in your discipline. Professional ethics and codes of responsibility insist on individual accountability. Where, then, are opportunities to learn from your experiences? When, and in what circumstances, can you reframe failure as a learning opportunity?

Case Study 2—Belmont House

Mary Jo Foley graduated from Lewiston University with a bachelor's degree in OT. She received her certification 6 months later and took a position with the St. Louis Pediatric Rehabilitation Center in the Children's Unit. While at the Pediatric Rehabilitation Center, Ms. Foley developed her skills as a member of the interdisciplinary team that worked together on a daily basis.

In 1997 Ms. Foley accepted a new position as an OT in a Family Support Program at St. Francis Hospital in Chicago. When she interviewed for the position, the program was designed as a 10-person inpatient unit with outpatient and community services provided on an as-needed basis. Six months after she began work at St. Francis, the Family Support Program changed focus and adopted an in-home family training model.

The program consisted of an OT, social worker, nutritionist, nurse, and speech pathologist. Each of these staff reported to the Family Support Program director for program direction and responsibility and to their own department for clinical and professional supervision. In keeping with the new community focus, the Family Support Program moved to an office building five blocks from the hospital. Ms. Foley's work world shifted from the hospital unit to the housing projects in the neighborhood. Rather than working with an interdisciplinary team in a predictable environment, Ms. Foley visited families as scheduled but never knew what to expect. As a professional, she felt unable to practice her OT skills because there were always intervening problems related to housing, family, or work. Ms. Foley felt unprepared to act as a social worker, housing coordinator, or employment specialist.

In addition, Ms. Foley felt removed from the OT department at the hospital. She shared an office with the Family Support Program's nurse and nutritionist, but she missed the ongoing clinical interaction with other therapists.

Ms. Foley has scheduled an appointment with you because you are the director of the department of OT. What advice would you offer to Ms. Foley concerning the opportunities for learning and leadership that this position offers? In addition, how would you help Ms. Foley reframe this situation? How would you analyze this situation from a human resource perspective? From a structural point of view?

References

Belasco, J. A., & Stayer, R. C. (1993). *Flight of the buffalo: Soaring to excellence, learning to let employees lead*. New York: Warner Books.

Bennis, W. (1989a). *On becoming a leader*. Reading, MA: Addison-Wesley Publishing Co.

Bennis, W. (1989b). *Why leaders can lead: The unconscious conspiracy continues*. San Francisco: Jossey-Bass Publishers.

Bennis, W. (1993). *An invented life: Reflections on leadership and change*. Reading, MA: Addison-Wesley Publishing Co.

Bennis, W., & Nanus, B. (1985). *Leaders: The strategies for taking charge*. New York: Harper and Row.

Bolman, L. G., & Deal, T. E. (1991). *Reframing organizations: Artistry, choice, and leadership*. San Francisco: Jossey-Bass Publishers.

Capra, F. (1982). *The turning point: Science, society, and the rising culture*. New York: Simon and Schuster.

Capra, F. (1991). *The tao of physics* (3rd ed.). Boston: Shambhala.

Covey, S. R. (1990). *The 7 habits of highly effective people: Powerful lessons in personal change*. New York: Simon and Schuster.

Daniels, S. (1991). *Disability paradigms compared*. Unpublished paper.

Deal, T .E., & Kennedy, A. A. (1982). *Corporate cultures: The rites and rituals of corporate life*. Reading, MA: Addison-Wesley Publishing Co.

DePree, M. (1989). *Leadership is an art*. New York: Doubleday.

Drucker, P. F. (1954). *The practice of management: A study of the most important function in American society*. New York: Harper and Row.

Huey, J. (1993, April 5). Managing in the midst of chaos. *Fortune*, 38-48.

Lewin, K. (1951). *Field theory in social science*. New York: Harper and Row.

Kouzes, J. M., & Posner, B. Z. (1987). *The leadership challenge: How to get extraordinary things done in organizations*. San Francisco: Jossey-Bass Publishers.

McLean, J. W., & Weitzel, W. (1991). *Leadership—Magic, myth, or method?* New York: American Management Association.

Senge, P. (1990). *The fifth discipline: The art & practice of the learning organization*. New York: Doubleday Currency.

Vail, P. B. (1989). *Managing as a performing art: New ideas for a world of chaotic change*. San Francisco: Jossey-Bass Publishers.

Wheatley, M. J. (1994). *Leadership and the new science: Learning about organization from an orderly universe*. San Francisco: Berrett-Koehler.

Wheatley, M. J., & Kellner-Rogers, M. (1996). *A simpler way*. San Francisco: Berrett-Koehler.

Wildavsky, A. (1984). *The nursing father: Moses as a political leader*. University, AL: The University of Alabama Press.

Wren, D. (1979). *The evolution of management thought*. New York: John Wiley and Sons.

Suggested Readings

Stogdill, R. M. (1974). *Handbook of leadership: A survey of theory and research*. New York: The Free Press.

Yukl, G. (1994). *Leadership in organizations* (3rd ed.) Englewood Cliffs, NJ: Prentice-Hall.

Answer Key

1. a
2. b
3. c
4. a
5. d
6. d
7. b
8. a
9. c
10. c

CHAPTER 3

Marketing Occupational Therapy Services

Karen Jacobs, EdD, OTR/L, CPE, FAOTA

Introduction

We are on the verge of an era when the needs for our services are so great as to push us to the brink of glory, if we can only deliver; or we may stumble, because we shall, I fear, cling tenaciously to what we have done without looking at what we might do if we were to take bold new directions. These were the words spoken by Cromwell in 1968. If the concept of marketing had been applied to the profession of OT 20 years ago, just imagine how much more of a significant role we may have been playing in the health care marketplace today.

The need for OT practitioners to have a good understanding of and apply the concepts of marketing has become more critical today. Marketing can play an important part in the success of an OT program and should become a familiar framework for the OT manager.

What Is Marketing?

Marketing has been a misunderstood term, most often used synonymously with public relations, selling, fundraising, or development. However, according to marketer Peter Drucker, "The aim of marketing is to make selling superfluous."

Marketing consists of meeting people's needs in the most efficient and therefore profitable manner (Cromwell, 1968). Kotler and Clarke (1987) define marketing in the following manner—marketing is the analysis, planning, implementation, and control of carefully formulated programs designed to bring about voluntary exchanges of values with target markets for the purpose of achieving organizational objectives. It relies heavily on designing the organization's offering in terms of the target markets' needs and desires, and on using effective pricing, communication, and distribution to inform, motivate, and service the markets.

Successful marketing planning begins with an idea that serves as the framework for all marketing efforts. It is an orientation that makes satisfying the customer's needs the integrating organizational principle. While the first impulse of the marketing novice is to design a program, such as a school-based work-related OT program, and then look for customers (e.g., adolescents with developmental disabilities), effective marketing dictates that the process be reversed. One first looks at the market and listens carefully to potential customers, and then designs the program to match the needs and desires of these potential customers.

Marketing Planning

The main benefits of marketing planning can be summarized as follows (Branch, 1962):

- Encourages systematic thinking ahead by management.
- Leads to better coordination of organizational efforts.
- Leads to the development of performance standards for control.
- Causes the organization to sharpen its guiding objectives and policies.
- Results in better preparedness for sudden developments.
- Brings about a more vivid sense in the participating managers of their interacting responsibilities.

Marketing planning can be viewed as a three-step process. Figure 3-1 delineates this process with planning as the first step. It encompasses identifying attractive markets, developing marketing strategies, and developing action programs. Execution is the second step. It includes carrying out the action programs. The third and final step involves marketing control. This final step requires measuring results, analyzing the causes of poor results, and taking corrective action. Adjustments in the plan, its execution, or both would include corrective actions that could be implemented.

Identifying Attractive Target Markets

Identifying the demands of the market is the first step in marketing. The market is defined as all actual or potential buyers of a product, service, or idea and can be considered in its entirety, such as all referral sources to an early intervention program, or divided into relevant segments according to variables, such as types of professionals (e.g., physicians, special education teachers, or nurses). Identifying attractive target markets includes the analysis of marketing opportunities. This analysis consists of:

- A self-audit
- Consumer analysis
- An analysis of other providers of similar services
- An environmental assessment

Self-Audit

A self-audit assesses the strengths, weaknesses, opportunities, and threats (SWOT analysis) of your department and/or specific program. Factors to be assessed may include:

- The reputation of your facility in the community
- The staff and their qualifications, such as a master's degree, certification as a hand therapist, or specialized training (e.g., neurodevelopmental treatment)
- Physical size of the program
- Location of the program (e.g., hospital/rehabilitation setting, community-based)
- Convenience of your location to mass transit, highways, and parking
- Type and quality of equipment
- Available budget
- Support from administration

This self-audit assists in understanding how well or poorly prepared you are to meet the marketplace demands. Ascertaining what you do well and maintaining that product (service) at an optimal level is part of marketing.

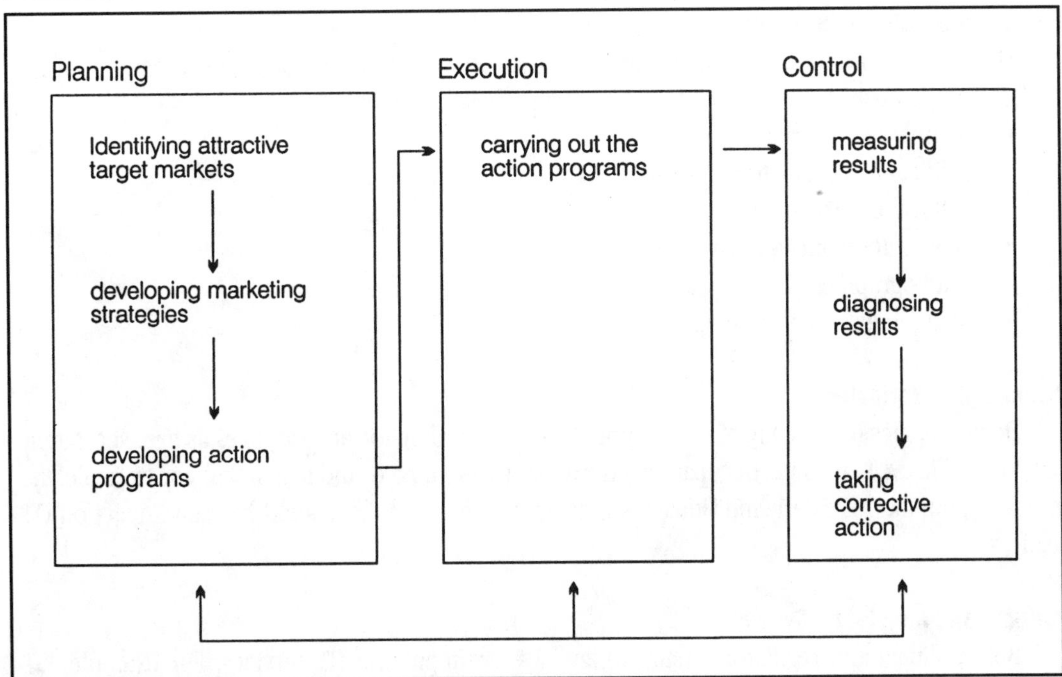

Figure 3-1. The marketing planning and control system.

Consumer Analysis

It is important to assess the potential consumers of your OT department's services within your catchment area. An analysis of some of the consumers who might use your products may include:

- Physicians
- Rehabilitation managers and consultants
- Nurses
- Vocational counselors
- Special education teachers
- Attorneys
- Administrators
- Workers with injuries
- Social workers
- Industrial companies
- Insurance companies
- Colleagues, such as other OTRs, COTAs, PTs

Analysis of Other Providers of Similar Services

How adequately the needs of the marketplace are being met, what areas are not being served, where duplication and overlap are occurring, and where opportunities for collaboration or joint venture exist can be ascertained through an analysis of other providers of similar services. One simple way to obtain information is to place your name on the mailing list of facilities/companies providing a similar product line. Reading through newsletters and brochures from the competition can be very insightful.

Environmental Assessment

The changes and trends that may have an impact on OT services and perhaps the future of the profession compose an environmental assessment. These include:

- Demographic variables
- Political and regulatory systems
- Cultural environment
- Economic/financial environment
- Psychographics
- Technological developments

Demographic Variables

Demographics is the study of human populations according to such variables as age, sex, family size, family life cycle, income, occupation, education, religion, race, and nationality. For example, the increasing number of elderly individuals is a demographic trend that should have an impact on OT services.

Political and Regulatory Systems

Both political and regulatory systems may have an impact on OT services. For example, OT programs located in Florida, Ohio, and Kentucky that are interested in developing work hardening programs will find that to receive reimbursement through their workers' compensation system, they will need to become accredited by the regulatory agency, the Commission on Accreditation of Rehabilitation Facilities (CARF), and adhere to CARF's Work Hardening Guidelines (CARF, 1991; Ellexson, 1989).

The implementation of the Americans With Disabilities Act (ADA) can have importance to the OT profession. OT practitioners can be advocates and assist in implementing the ADA which provides comprehensive civil rights protection from discrimination in employment, transportation, public accommodations, telecommunications, and the activities of state and local government for individuals with disabilities. For example, Title 1—Employment provides the OT with the opportunity to provide post-offer screenings and devise reasonable accommodations so that the individual with a disability can perform the essential functions of the job (ADA, 1991).

Cultural Environment

Culture is a force that affects individuals within society's behaviors, values, perceptions, preferences, and behaviors. The United States is becoming a more multicultural society, and it becomes imperative that OT practitioners develop an understanding and sensitivity to the culture profiles of clients within their catchment area. Having practitioners who are bilingual can be most beneficial and may be the variable that assists in making a product successful.

Economic/Financial Environment

An analysis of the economic/financial environment revealed that the following factors may have a positive impact for OT services (Gilfoyle, 1988):

- Eight percent of the gross national product is spent on programs that support dependency.
- One in five American adults suffers from some type of disability.
- Over $45 billion a year is spent on workers' compensation.

- Ten percent of corporation expenditures is spent on health care.
- Approximately 300,000 students with disabilities who graduate each year from high schools are unemployed.

Psychographics

Psychographics is the technique of measuring consumers' social class, lifestyle, and personality characteristics and can provide information on activities, interests, and opinions of these individuals. Understanding the psychographic profile of your consumers might provide information to assist in strategizing a product to them.

Technological Developments

The technology arena is greatly advancing and will have an impact on the type of high-tech evaluation and treatment equipment available to OT programs. As computers become more commonplace in OT departments, these technological advances will allow for information to be exchanged in a more efficient manner. For example, many programs send instantaneous reports to insurance companies within 24 hours via a computer modem or communicate worldwide in a matter of seconds through a facsimile machine.

Selecting Target Markets and Market Segments

Once analysis is completed, there are three steps in target marketing. Market segmentation refers to the act of dividing a market into distinct groups of buyers who might require separate products and marketing mixes. For example, physicians can be segmented into pediatricians or neurologists; allied health professionals can be segmented into speech pathologists and PTs. Market targeting is the act of evaluating and selecting one or more of the markets to enter. An example of this is targeting orthopedic surgeons as the main referral source for a hand therapy program. Product positioning is the act of formulating a competitive position for the product and a detailed marketing mix.

Developing Marketing Strategies

Developing marketing strategies includes the development of objectives for each identified target market and their implementation. The four P's—product, place, price, and promotion—are the strategies that can be used to influence the demand for a product. Here is how each of these "P's" is used is the marketing mix (Clopton, 1986; Jacobs, 1987).

Product

Simply stated, what we do as OT practitioners are our products. That is, OT assists individuals to become as independent as possible.

Ideally, the goal is to offer a product line—a variety of products associated with one another by an overall theme. For example, an OT department may have an industrial rehabilitation program whose product line includes post-offer screening, baseline evaluation, job capacity evaluation, occupational capacity evaluation, work capacity evaluation, ergonomic consultation, and work hardening. A school-based OT department may offer a product line of sensory integration evaluation and treatment, work-related assessment and programming, and classroom consultation.

How a product is packaged may influence its success. It is important to make sure all your paperwork (e.g., brochures and evaluation write-ups) have a professional appearance. The ability to access information quickly and be able to present it in a professional manner to the target markets is an asset.

Many new product ideas are generated by understanding our client's needs and wants through direct surveys, projective tests, focus group discussions, and letters and complaints received. It is important to note that for every unhappy customer, you lose 50 others, and that 80% of your business is coming from 20% of your customers (Baum & Luebben, 1986).

Place

OT services can be provided in a variety of places. Some of these include:

- Free-standing facilities located in professional buildings, industrial parks, and shopping centers
- Free-standing facilities affiliated with outpatient service departments, rehabilitation centers, or hospitals
- As part of a comprehensive rehabilitation or acute care facility/program/hospital
- At work site programs provided by a company to serve the needs of a specific business or industry
- Schools
- Nursing homes

When analyzing the place aspect of marketing planning, other variables that should be considered are the hours the program is offered for business. For example, is your program open during hours convenient to your markets or your staff? An innovative aspect of place could be the provision of day care services for the children and/or elderly patients of clients who are attending your program.

Price

The price or fee schedule for OT services (products) should be based on cost, competitive factors, geographic area, and what the consumer is willing to pay. It is important for the price to be commensurate with perceived value (Jacobs, 1987).

Promotion

Promotion is the vehicle of communicating information to your markets about the product's merits, place, and price. Instruments of promotion are advertising, sales promotion, publicity, and personal selling.

Advertising

Advertising involves the use of a paid message presented in a recognized medium and by an identified sponsor, with the purpose to inform, persuade, and remind. Some advertising vehicles include:

- Printed ads—found in newspapers, journals, and magazines
- Brochures
- Direct mail
- Broadcasts
- Transits
- Billboards
- Quarterly newsletters

Sales Promotion

Sales promotion is the use of a wide variety of short-term incentives to encourage purchase of the product. This approach is most effective when used in conjunction with advertising. For example, at an open house for an industrial rehabilitation program, a successful sales promotion technique used to increase new referrals was a business card drawing for "service certificates" good for a day's worth of work hardening or work evaluation on any new referrals.

Publicity

Publicity is often described as a marketing stepchild because it is relatively underused in relation to the real contribution it can make (Kotler, 1983b). The most positive aspect of publicity is that it is free. However, one has little control over the placement of it and thus it becomes difficult to focus publicity on specific target markets. An example of publicity might be to contact the local media, through a press release, about an upcoming event at your facility (e.g., activities to celebrate OT month). Perhaps if the media finds your event newsworthy and they are not understaffed, they will send a reporter to cover the event. Whether or not the reporter writes a story can be dependent on variables out of your control, such as available time and space in the newspaper. However, a successful strategy in utilizing publicity more effectively has been to develop a rapport with the media. Personally contact your local newspaper and radio station and introduce yourself; let them know about your program and offer to be available to them if they need a resource.

Personal Selling

Face-to-face communication between you and your audience is the most effective form of promotion. It is, however, the most expensive. It is also the method most used by OT practitioners (Jacobs, 1987). Word-of-mouth recommendations by staff and consumers of an OT program (products) are a powerful sales pitch. Other successful personal selling methods include the following:

- Exhibiting at various conferences
- Developing a free speakers' bureau
- Presenting inservice training to physicians and OT and physical therapy (PT) practitioners
- Presenting continuing education workshops
- Lecturing
- Attending professional meetings for various organizations
- Holding an open house
- Holding continuing education seminars for referral sources

Focus groups have been found to be an effective marketing technique. These techniques use primary referral sources, such as physicians, to provide feedback on current programming efforts and recommendations for future program modifications. The use of focus groups allows the manager to quickly incorporate modifications perceived to be important by the referral sources. This in turn should generate an increased commitment on the part of the referral sources to the program.

Focus Group Interviewing

Focus group interviewing is becoming one of the major marketing research tools for gaining insight into consumer thoughts and feelings (Kotler, 1983a). Focus group interviewing consists of inviting 6 to 10 participants to spend a few hours with a skilled interviewer to discuss any designated subject matter, such as the feasibility of developing a school-based OT work program. Focus group practitioners are usually paid a small sum for attending the meeting. These are typically held in pleasant surroundings, with refreshments served. The interview begins with broad questions, such as "What do you think about OT work programming for elementary school-aged students with special needs?" leading to focusing in on more specific questions on the subject matter such as "What do you think about the feasibility of an OT work program being established at Butler Elementary School?" The interviewer encourages free and easy discussion among participants, hoping that the group dynamics will bring out deep feelings and thoughts (Kotler & Clarke, 1984). Although the results cannot be generalizable to the market as a whole due to its small sample size, the information gathered can provide insight into participants' perceptions, attitudes, and satisfaction. Information obtained can help define what issues need to be researched more formally or may provide the foundation for being able to develop a product which will meet the consumer's needs (Kotler & Clarke, 1984).

Execution of the Marketing Plan

Once you have selected your target market, develop a specific marketing mix (product, price, place, and promotion) for your market which stresses the benefits of your product(s). When executing action programs, a timeline should be delineated, such as a 12-month period, to measure whether objectives and goals are being met. The action plan should be dynamic and be able to be changed throughout the year as new opportunities and problems arise. Ideally, actions should be assigned to specific individuals who are given exact completion dates. An action that might be assigned to a staff therapist can include developing a single paragraph description of the sensory integration program provided by the OT department. The therapist is given a 1-week timeline to complete this action. Once the description is completed, the manager has 2 weeks to incorporate this information into a brochure being developed to promote the expanded product line of pediatric OT to potential referral sources. In this case, as in all aspects of promotion, it is important to communicate in a language that is familiar to your market. Avoid professional jargon!

Marketing Control

Marketing is an area where rapid obsolescence of objectives, policies, strategies, and programs is a constant possibility (Kotler & Clarke, 1984). Marketing control attempts to circumvent this dilemma and assists in maximizing the probability that a product will achieve its short- and long-term objectives. It is important to measure program results, diagnose these results, and take corrective action, if necessary. There are three types of marketing control (Kotler & Clarke, 1984):

1. **Annual plan control** consists of the steps used during the year to monitor and correct deviations from the marketing plan to ensure that annual sales and profit goals are being achieved.
2. **Profitability control** refers to the efforts used to determine the actual profit or loss of different marketing entities such as the products (services) or market segments.
3. **Strategic control** is a systematic evaluation of the organization's market performance in relation to the current and forecasted marketing environment.

Unfortunately, as uncommon as marketing planning is in health care organizations, marketing control is even less common. If health care organizations do bother to evaluate performance, it is usually limited to clinical evaluation: "We provided a (clinically) good service." In the process of providing these services, however, health care organizations are often squandering scarce resources, unaware of which resources are being productively used and which are being wasted (Kotler & Clarke, 1984).

Conclusion

A bright future can be a certainty for therapists who are prepared to accept the reality of today's and tomorrow's health care environment. It will be increasingly competitive, with various professions vying for control of the patient and, thereby, the dollars. It will be increasingly complex. It will be increasingly controlled by payers—government, insurers, and corporations (Pickelle & Ramos, 1991).

Therapists' abilities to market—yes, market—their skills and knowledge to those that control the dollars will be an ever-present requirement for success. It will likely make the difference between encroachment by other professions and a resulting second-class specialty, and a proud and effective profession placed squarely in a leadership position within the health care industry (Pickelle & Ramos, 1991).

We need to rally to this cheer! Marketing should guide the OT practitioner in his or her role as a manager in the marketplace. Having access to an expert in marketing to assist in the development of a marketing plan would be the ideal situation, but this is not always the case. On the other hand, the worst possible scenario would be one where even an informal market analysis does not precede program development. If this is the case for you, a word of caution: remember that designing a program and then looking for customers typically leads to facing an uphill battle to success. At the very least, before investing a great deal of useless time, effort, and money, attempt to perform a market analysis on your own following the guidelines presented in this chapter and in other available literature.

Questions

1. Peter Drucker describes the aim of marketing as:
   a. Making selling superfluous
   b. Maximizing sales
   c. Obtaining the highest price on your product
   d. Developing the largest size product line

2. A market is:
   a. All actual or potential buyers of a product, service, or idea
   b. A place
   c. A price
   d. Transactions between two buyers of a product

3. The technique of interviewing a selected group of individuals is called:
   a. Task group interviewing
   b. Activity analysis
   c. Strategic marketing interviewing
   d. Focus group interviewing

4. Which of the following is a false statement regarding the benefits of marketing planning?
    a. Encourages systematic thinking
    b. Results in better preparedness for sudden development
    c. Leads to better coordination of an organization's efforts
    d. Leads to the development of poorer performance standards for control

5. An individual's lifestyle is measured by the technique called:
    a. Cognitive analysis
    b. Psychographics
    c. Life cycle analysis
    d. Lifestyle

6. The most common promotion technique used by OTs is:
    a. Advertising
    b. Personal selling
    c. Sales promotion
    d. Publicity

7. What is not a type of marketing control?
    a. Annual plan control
    b. Profitability control
    c. Strategic control
    d. Segment marketing control

8. Which are the three steps in target marketing?
    a. Market segmentation, market targeting, product positioning
    b. Market segmentation, market targeting, price positioning
    c. Product positioning, price targeting, market segmentation
    d. Market targeting, market pricing, target place

9. The four P's of the marketing mix are:
    a. Price, packaging, place, promotion
    b. Place, price, promotion, product
    c. Product, packaging, promotion, place
    d. Product, procedure, price, packaging

10. The three-step process for marketing planning and control is:
    a. Planning, execution, control
    b. Control, execution, planning
    c. Execution, planning, control
    d. Planning, control, execution

Case Study 1

The sole OT in a private school for students ages 5 to 21 with learning disabilities wants to expand her product line to include work assessment and programming. After approaching the school's administrator about this idea, she is told that she must first develop a marketing plan to support the feasibility of such a venture. The therapist approached this task as a three-step process: planning, execution, and control.

Step One: Planning

Within planning there are three steps: identifying attractive markets, developing marketing strategies, and developing action programs. The first step was to identify target markets and consisted of: a self-audit, consumer analysis, an analysis of other providers of similar services, and an environmental assessment.

- **Self-Audit.** In performing a self-audit the following strengths were revealed: there was both physical space for expansion of the program and enough funds for the purchase of specialized supplies and equipment, and the OT had an excellent reputation within the school.
- **Consumer Analysis.** Although the therapist wanted to provide work assessment and programming to the complete student market, she narrowed her focus and targeted those learning disabled students ages 12 to 21 years.
- **Other Providers of Similar Services.** There were no other providers of similar services; however, academic programming utilized a functional curriculum approach that might provide the opportunity for future collaboration.
- **Environmental Assessment.** The catchment area for the school was 80 communities providing for a large cross-section of students. In addition, the school itself was located in an upper-middle class community among many service industries.

The second step within planning is to develop marketing strategies. The four P's—product, price, place, and promotion—were analyzed as follows:

- **Product.** Work assessments, work programming, and classroom consultation with teachers.
- **Price.** The charge for OT already has been incorporated into the total school tuition.
- **Place.** Programming will be located in various areas: local stores, classrooms, school cafeterias, and OT treatment areas.
- **Promotion.** The therapist will provide inservice training to teachers on the program, devise a display for the school corridor with photographs of students in work OT, and contact a local newspaper to write an article about the program.

Developing an action plan requires the correct marketing mix.

Step Two: Execution

Step Three: Control

Once the program has been executed, the third step will be to monitor whether the program is meeting its goal and objectives. This would be a dynamic process, where changes would be made and the three-step process would begin again.

Case Study 2

There are seven OTs in a hand therapy clinic that is part of and located in an acute care hospital. Industrial rehabilitation, particularly work hardening, has become the new "buzz words" in OT, and the OT department would like to begin to include this aspect of practice into its product line. As director of the OT department, you decide to perform a market analysis to ascertain the feasibility of expanding your product line to include industrial rehabilitation.

Your first step is to identify attractive target markets. In identifying these markets, the analysis of marketing opportunities should be performed. In this case the analysis consists of: a self-audit, consumer analysis, an analysis of other providers of similar services, and an environmental assessment.

A self-audit of the OT department consists of analyzing its strengths, weaknesses, opportunities, and threats (SWOT analysis). For example, some strengths might include:

- Seven master's degree level OTs.
- Three of these therapists have specialized training and certification as hand therapists.
- Both the hospital and the OT department have an excellent reputation in the community.
- The hospital is conveniently located near mass transit and major highways and has attached parking.

The analysis might reveal the following weaknesses:

- Limited physical space within the department for expansion.
- Limited financial resources for the purchase of new equipment.

The following opportunities might be revealed:

- The hospital recently purchased an office building in close proximity to the hospital and all available space has not been allocated.
- Funding would be available for programs being housed in this new facility.

At present, the aspect thought to be a threat is that the available space in the new freestanding facility would be assigned to a department other than OT.

A consumer analysis reveals the following markets as potential users of the industrial rehabilitation program:

- Physicians
- Workers with injuries
- Nurses
- Local industry
- Insurance companies
- Rehabilitation managers and consultants
- Attorneys
- Colleagues, such as other OTRs

An analysis of other providers of similar services revealed that there were no industrial rehabilitation programs in any other acute care hospital or outpatient rehabilitation facility within a 30-mile radius of the hospital.

Finally, an environmental assessment indicated that the hospital was located in a lower-middle class, blue-collar community, with construction being the predominate industry.

Once the analysis was completed, market segmentation was performed. That is, the potential consumers of the industrial rehabilitation program were divided into distinct groups. For example, physicians were segmented into orthopedic surgeons and neurologists. This market was targeted further by selecting only the orthopedic surgeons as the main referral source for the industrial rehabilitation program.

Developing marketing strategies specific to each targeted market is the next step in the analysis. In this case, the director decided to start with the orthopedic surgeons as the primary market. At this point, the director enlisted the assistance of the hospital's marketing department. Working together, they devised the four P's. The product, an industrial rehabilitation program, was divided into a product line that included: work capacity evaluation, work hardening, job analysis, and preplacement screening. The industrial rehabilitation program would be located (the place) in the newly acquired free-standing office building owned by the hospital. The price for the program would continue to be regulated by the hospital's fee schedule. Promotion was handled through the marketing department of the hospital, who would advertise the industrial rehabilitation program in the orthopedic surgeons' quarterly newsletter and in its monthly professional journal, develop brochures, and send direct mailings to these physicians. The publicity used to promote the industrial rehabilitation program to orthopedic surgeons would be through articles in the hospital's monthly newsletter and human interest stories that would focus on an individual client's successful return to work. Additional stories could be covered by the local community newspaper. Finally, the OTs would become directly involved with personal selling by holding an open house for the orthopedic surgeons and providing a presentation of the industrial rehabilitation program at the monthly physician's breakfast.

Once the industrial rehabilitation program was in place, it would be analyzed on a 6-month basis to determine that program goals and objectives were being met.

References

Americans with Disabilities Act. (1991, July 26). *Federal Register*.

Baum, C. M., & Luebben, A. J. (1986). *Prospective payment systems: A handbook for health care clinicians*. Thorofare, NJ: SLACK Incorporated.

Branch, M. (1962). *The corporate planning process*. New York: American Management Association.

Clopton, D. (1986, May 14). Marketing occupational therapy. *Occupational Therapy Forum, 15*, 19.

Commission on Accreditation of Rehabilitation Facilities. (1991). *Standards manual for organizations serving people with disabilities*. Tucson, AZ: Author.

Cromwell, F. (1968). American Occupational Therapy Association.

Ellexson, M. (1989). *Work hardening. In work programs guidelines*. Rockville, MD: American Occupational Therapy Association.

Gilfoyle, E. (1988, August 22). Gilfoyle urges promotion of OT during AOTA conference ceremony. *OT Week, 1*, 31.

Jacobs, K. (1987, May). Marketing occupational therapy. *Am J Occup Ther, 41*(5), 315-320.

Kotler, P. (1983a). *Principles of marketing* (2nd ed.). Englewood Cliffs, NJ: Prentice-Hall.

Kotler, P. (1983b). *Principles of marketing—Instructor's manual with cases*. Englewood Cliffs, NJ: Prentice-Hall.

Kotler, P., & Clarke, R. (1984). *Marketing management* (5th ed.). Englewood Cliffs, NJ: Prentice-Hall.

Kotler, P., & Clarke, R. (1987). *Marketing for health care organizations*. Englewood Cliffs, NJ: Prentice-Hall.

Pickelle, C., & Ramos, T. (1991, February/March). Publishers' message. *Rehab Management*, 9.

Suggested Readings

Hershman, A. G. (1984). Reimbursement in private practice. *Am J Occup Ther, 38*(5), 299-306.

LaCroix, E. (1987, October 30). *Setting up and surviving a private practice*. Bedford, MA: Massachusetts Association for Occupational Therapy, Annual Conference.

Marketing occupational therapy services. (1984, August). *Occupational Therapy Newspaper,* 4.

Occupational therapy benefits from CARF changes. (1987). *Occupational Therapy News, 41*, 1.

Olson, T., & Urban, C. (1985). Marketing. In J. Bair & M. Gray (Eds.). *The occupational therapy manager.* Rockville, MD: American Occupational Therapy Association.

Richardson, J. E. (Ed.). (1987). *Marketing 87/88*. Gullford, CT: The Dushkin Publishing Group, Inc.

Scott, S., & Dennis, D. (Eds.). (1988). *Payment for occupational therapy services*. Rockville, MD: American Occupational Therapy Association.

Answer Key

1. a
2. a
3. d
4. d
5. b
6. b
7. d
8. a
9. b
10. a

CHAPTER 4

Cost Management

Martha K. Logigian, MS, OTR/L

Introduction

The health care market continues to evolve from a fee-for-service (FFS) environment common prior to the 1980s to the current process of managed care. Industry officials believe that this evolution will continue until we reach a level of managed competition (Table 4-1). As practitioners we must be aware of the changes, knowledgeable of the processes they encompass, and possess the skills to successfully negotiate them including that OT is a covered service in health care benefit packages. In addition, health care charges and expenditures have risen at an accelerated rate creating serious cash flow problems (Coddington, Palmquist, & Trollinger, 1985). Change in reimbursement is unavoidable as health care institutions and professionals are under pressure by insurance companies and the government to conserve. In the past the key to an institution's success was increasing revenue, often achieved through increasing volume. However, critical shifts have occurred as concerns about cost have intensified. This has led to a refocus on evaluating the cost and effectiveness of any intervention (Woolhandler & Himmelstein, 1989). This analysis of cost and benefit is critical to the future of successful financial management.

Prospective Payment

In the 1980s, the Social Security Amendment was enacted to limit hospital spending. This established a prospective payment system (PPS) for hospital care, eliminating the FFS practice in place for many years. Under a PPS system, hospital discharges were classified in diagnosis-related groups (DRGs). Assignment to a DRG was based on diagnosis, age, sex, co-morbidities, procedure, and discharge status. The DRG-based method pays a fixed amount for a period of hospitalization regardless of its duration or intensity of care. The reimbursement for a specific patient is determined by the average cost for the particular disorder or DRG and, except in unusual cases, is unaffected by the costs actually incurred in treating the patient (Vladeck, 1984). Special consideration is given to cases referred to as outliers and those transferred between hospitals. Outliers are cases with either extremely long lengths of stay, labeled day outliers, or extraordinarily high costs, labeled cost outliers. Because an institution's reimbursement is based on prospective fixed rates, it is at risk for costs exceeding the DRG rate, yet stands to gain if costs do not exceed expenses. At present, this system includes most Medicare inpatient services, excluding psychiatric, non-acute, and children's

Table 4-1
Evolution of the Health Care Market

Managed Competition: A theory that suggests that the individual employee receive a fixed sum from the employer and chooses a health plan. If the plan chosen costs more than the employer's fixed sum, the employee is responsible for the difference. The individual employee would have a tax incentive to select the lower priced options because he or she would only be able to deduct the amount of the lowest cost option. The proposal's proponents believe this would encourage individual consumers to be more price conscious and would cause health care insurers to hold down the cost of their plans to make them more competitive. Because insurance under this proposed system is not tied to the employer, employees would not lose coverage when they change jobs. Under this proposed system there is no provision to set premiums that appropriately cover the risk of an individual patient or specific patient population. Since originally introduced, the term has come to be used also for purchasers contracting with an integrated system to provide comprehensive services to their enrollees.

↑

Capitation: The per capita payment for providing a specific menu of health services to a defined population over a set period of time. The provider usually receives, in advance, a negotiated monthly payment. This payment is the same regardless of the amount of service rendered.

↑

Risk: The chance or possibility of loss. For example, physicians may be held at risk if hospitalization rates exceed agreed-upon thresholds. The sharing of risk is often employed as a resource utilization mechanism. Risk is also defined in insurance terms as the probability of loss associated with a given population.

↑

Pricing Package: Special prices given for a collection of specific services or benefits the organization is obligated to provide under terms of its contracts with subscriber groups or individuals.

↑

Contracted Discounting: Individual employers or business coalitions seek a discounted contract directly with providers for health care services with no HMO/PPO intermediary. This enables the employer to include in the plan the specific services preferred by the employees.

↑

Discounted Fees: Physician's services are provided as fee-for-service but at a negotiated rate less than the usual fee.

↑

Fee-for-Services: The patient is charged according to a fee schedule set for each service or procedure provided. The total bill will vary by the number of services/procedures actually received. The patient is billed at the time of service.

Adapted from *Glossary of terms used in managed care*. Medical Group Management Association, 104 Inverness Terrace East, Englewood, CO 80112. © 1997.

hospital-based services (Heinemamum, 1988). However, it appears imminent that some type of DRG-based system will be used for non-acute services.

Health Care Changes

However, since the late 1980s it has been clear that these changes were not adequate to control health care costs. Thus, other alternative delivery systems (ADSs) developed in response to the continued demand to reduce costs. ADSs usually involve a significant integration between payer and payee with the payer managing the care. Health maintenance organizations (HMOs) and preferred provider organizations (PPOs) (*The Preferred Provider Organization*, 1984) were the major types at this time. An HMO is a prepaid organized delivery system where the organization and primary care physicians (PCPs) assume some financial risk for the care provided to its enrolled members. Often the HMO physicians are paid on a capitated basis.

A PPO acts as a broker between the purchaser of care and the provider. Consumers are encouraged by incentives (or disincentives, i.e., extra fees and benefits) to use the providers from the plan. Currently, ADSs are evolving into integrated delivery systems (IDSs), which also include exclusive provider organizations (EPOs) and full risk capitation. In an EPO, the patient must use the providers from the plan. Capitation is a system of predetermined, fixed reimbursement for a defined set of services for designated individuals. Under a typical capitation arrangement, each enrollee is assigned to a specific provider who receives a flat payment per assigned enrollee per month. The provider is required to provide or arrange for all covered medical services for the assigned enrollee (Palmer, 1996).

Under all of these systems, care is typically "managed" and driven by PCPs as gatekeepers or coordinators of services (Table 4-2). Managed care refers to this process, which is in contrast to the traditional unmanaged FFS care. Some traditional FFS providers continue in indemnity health insurance plans, but even here they are often controlled by a case manager or third party administrator for the company.

In the past, the controls used to manage a patient's care commonly included pre-admission certification, limitations on length of stay through utilization review, mandatory second opinion prior to surgery, and non-physician case managers coordinating the care process for consumers. Now the focus is on the coordination of the continuum of care in an effort to further control cost while at the same time ensuring efficiencies (*Viewpoints*, 1996).

This concept involves an integrated system of care that guides and tracks enrollees (i.e., covered lives) over time through a comprehensive array of health services spanning all levels of care. Consumers are seeking to join health care programs that provide this continuum via one-stop shopping for all health care services. If these services are under a single payment mechanism, all the better.

Employers are looking for HMOs and PPOs that offer low prices for health care services, assuming the enrollees stay within the network to select physician, hospital, and other health care services. To the extent that an organization offers a comprehensive, cost-effective continuum of care, it can establish attractive programs for third party payers. Under capitation, there can be additional risk sharing which has intensified the process. In a gatekeeper plan, specialist and hospital care can be delivered only with the gatekeeper's approval. The gatekeeper is placed at financial risk for specialist referral and hospital care that often serves as a disincentive. In many cases the insurance plan continues to share in the financial losses (downside risk) and gains (upside risk) with the providers. The providers (e.g., PCPs and hospitals) may also share risk among each other through mechanisms for risk sharing such as incentive pools, limits on gains or losses, and minimum reimbursement levels.

When the gatekeeper does not share risk, the gatekeeper is paid separately for this service which is viewed as case management. The IDSs, particularly state Medicaid programs, purchase these services. In managed competition, IDSs buy the entire primary care network (PCN) to better control the process.

Today, large IDSs provide care for thousands of covered lives. From the point when members are enrolled, they manage services of the continuum from outreach, health promotion, and housing to ambulatory, acute, extended, and home care (Evashwick, 1989). They are overseen by administrators, with PCPs controlling access to the system. Case managers, also referred to as care coordinators, facilitate collaboration among clinicians and direct service providers. This ensures high quality, cost-effective care by arranging the variety of services appropriate to meet the needs of the patient at a given time and efficiently changing these services as the patient's needs change (Evashwick, 1989).

The challenge under a capitated reimbursement arrangement is to provide high quality, cost-effective care while meeting the overall goal of reducing the cost of providing health care services. At the same time, outcomes must be maintained or improved. The incentive to perform well under a capitated arrangement is the opportunity to increase one's net revenue by reaping the savings accrued from cost reduction (Lanute, 1994). In other words, the provider is paid a fixed amount

Table 4-2
To Successfully Manage a Capitated Full-Risk Member Population, an Organization Must Change Its Focus

Old Paradigm	New Paradigm
Patient Model	Member Model
Illness/Curative Model	Wellness/Preventive Model
Tracking Beds and Admits	Tracking Outcomes and Health Status
Service Use Earns Money	Service Use Costs Money

Adapted from Sharp Consulting Institute, 8665 Gibbs Drive, Suite 200, San Diego, CA 92123.

regardless of the services performed, so the greater the cost-effectiveness of the services provided, the greater the savings. Providers are cognizant of the need to provide adequate care as they want to prevent worse problems from occurring later or enrollee dissatisfaction resulting in leaving the system to seek care elsewhere.

In today's reimbursement market, it is imperative to know the costs related to managing a business. In addition, payers are looking for hospitals to shorten lengths of stay, reduce unnecessary service utilization, emphasize outpatient vs. more costly inpatient care, decrease expensive high-tech interventions, and offer deep price discounts. These cost-driven dynamics will be amplified by changes at the federal level once national health care reform becomes a reality. If fact, the recent federal deficit-reduction plan contains deep cuts in what the government will pay for Medicare or Medicaid.

In response to these pressures, health care institutions and providers have been forced to change the way they do business. Institutions are launching multi-year plans which focus on diversification and enhancement of preferred provider relationships to position themselves in regional and national marketplaces. Individual and small group providers are joining larger networks to enhance their chance of survival in highly competitive markets. Acquisitions and mergers are now commonplace as they enable cuts in expenses by stressing economies of scale (Shields & Young, 1992).

To further improve net revenue, institutions are eliminating duplication, downsizing workforces, encouraging cross-training of health professionals, and increasing productivity (Vasquez, 1996). Although thousands of hospital beds have been closed nationwide, payers continue to demand deep price discounts which force hospitals to make further cuts such as shorter lengths of stay, reduction in ancillary service utilization, and decreases in the use of expensive high-tech interventions. There has been a shift from the use of expensive acute rehabilitation hospitals for patients needing extended care to sub-acute rehabilitation programs and skilled nursing facilities (SNFs) that are believed to be more cost-effective. This is particularly so if the sub-acute and SNF programs are under the control of the insurer—costs can be monitored more closely.

In the 1980s, emphasis was on ambulatory care rather than more costly inpatient care. Now it is shifting to wellness and health promotion while limiting access to ambulatory visits and procedures (Goldsmith, 1989). For example, in the past a person with chronic back pain could pursue individual therapy sessions including the use of modalities to manage the pain. Now, reimbursers are approving a therapy assessment and back school program. The patient is responsible for charges beyond this pre-approved plan.

Some recently proposed changes to Medicare are the result of the Balanced Budget Act of 1997. The American Occupational Therapy Association (AOTA) has advocated for a variety of issues including the most recent from the Health Care Financing Administration's (HCFA's) proposed changes for 1999 Medicare physician's fee schedule. These include changes for OT as an outpatient service. Among the proposed changes OT will be codified as a distinctive service as is PT, and practice expenses will be based on relative value units (RVUs). Changes in Medicare and other payers will continue to evolve as health care financing moves toward managed capitation. It is critical for managers to have up-to-date knowledge of these changes. One means of remaining in the know is to keep in touch with AOTA via their website (www.AOTA.org).

As clinical procedures and services are streamlined, providers must not lose sight that patient satisfaction and outcome will influence choice in this new marketplace. Care must be measured from the patient's perspective as this is critical to financial success in managed care markets. To achieve patient satisfaction, providers are seeking ways to influence positive outcome. Through interdisciplinary care improvement teams, health professionals address such issues as patient flow, the discharge process, patient outreach, and promotion and cost-efficiencies. Teams such as these may develop critical pathways to improve quality and cut costs. Pathways are standardized treatment protocols which provide an optimal sequencing of interventions by members of the health care team for a specific diagnosis designed to minimize delays and resource utilization. At the same time they carefully outline the limitations of a program to avoid duplication of effort and economies of utilization. For example, prior to surgery for a total hip replacement, a PT visits the patient's home to teach the patient how to use crutches and carry out an exercise program. If it is apparent that durable medical equipment may be needed, this is noted in the record.

On day 3 of the path, the OT automatically performs a safety evaluation to determine what specific equipment is needed for a safe discharge home. The equipment is ordered to be delivered to the patient's home on the day of discharge. This eliminates the need for a specific referral to OT for the assessment and facilitates an efficient discharge. In addition, the hospital stay is shortened as paperwork and delays are reduced, and the patient returns home with home care follow-up, avoiding a costly rehab hospital stay. The efficiencies enable cost savings as well as patient satisfaction.

Budgets

In today's reimbursement market, it is imperative to know the costs related to managing a business. In addition, once the costs are known a budget must be formulated to control and manage expenses. A budget in OT typically focuses on two major areas: capital budget and operations budget.

A capital budget typically includes items and renovations that cost above a fixed amount (e.g., a purchase value or cost of $250 or more) and has a life of 2 years or more. These include buildings, major renovations, and equipment such as a fluidotherapy unit. Capital budgeting is usually completed once a year. The process involves completing requests (Table 4-3) which are submitted to the administration for consideration for funding. Capital items are viewed separately by funding agencies with consideration for depreciation and possible tax credits, which is why separate budgeting for these items occurs.

An operations budget reflects day-to-day financial activity of an area. It commonly includes timely information on volume, personnel and nonpersonnel expenses, and revenue. It is prepared yearly, usually 6 to 8 months prior to the beginning of the fiscal year. Table 4-4 is an example of a cost accounting report used to form an operational budget for each department in an acute care hospital. This type of report provides monthly statements of financial activity of the area/depart-

Table 4-3
Capital Equipment Budget Request
Fiscal Year

I.	**Item**	Description Vender Quantity Unit cost Shipping Installation Charge to cost center
II.	**Type**	Brand new item Replacement item More of existing item
III.	**Justification**	(What problem are you trying to solve?) FTE, space, supply
IV.	**Impacts**	Financial (1) Expenses—one time, ongoing (2) Revenue—volume, charge Other
V.	**Consequence of Not Having This**	
VI.	**Rank Order (Within Your Department)**	

ment. Actual refers to the amount spent, volume completed, or revenue obtained for that month. The term budget is the amount budgeted for the month that is based on a yearly figure divided by 12 months. Monthly budget reports are provided to each area/department with detailed information on expenditures and revenue. These reports present the budgeted amount, actual costs, and variance that is the difference between the two. Negative variance is demonstrated with brackets around the numbers while positive variance has no brackets.

Volume is presented as the workload unit designated for the area. For OT, a common unit of measure is time or visits. To determine this, a productivity system is useful. Productivity is a critical factor in controlling cost and meeting volume projections (Marqulies & Duval, 1984; Orefice & Jennings, 1984). In a therapy department, it involves establishing service requirements for the amount of direct care expected to be provided per therapist per day, i.e., frequency and intensity of services provided and the effect on resource utilization (Logigian, 1987). Questions that should be answered when productivity is considered include: Can therapy programs be done in groups? What equipment is absolutely essential for the patient? Should evening hours be established for outpatients and those patients admitted to the hospital late in the day? Are referrals prioritized and handled in an efficient manner? What is the appropriate number of direct and indirect patient/client contact hours for therapists?

To help determine staff productivity, one method is a time-based analysis, such as in Table 4-5. The information on this table represents data collected from patient charges. One unit is equal to 15 minutes of direct patient contact and a non-time based unit indicates the use of a modality. Charge slips which are batched and submitted daily to an institution's charge and audit department list services provided for each treatment. This information is utilized for patient billing and development of a productivity report.

To identify an appropriate productivity measure, a regional survey provides information on comparable departments. Unique variables and constraints can be considered such as transporta-

Table 4-4
Cost Accounting Report
Cost Center

1. **Workload Unit**
   Units of treatment
2. **Total Personnel (FTEs)**
   Actual = All hours paid (productive and nonproductive) as reflected in position control report
   Budget = Total hours as reflected in staff plan
3. **Employee Benefit Expense**
   Allocated portion of benefits contribution made by the hospital as determined by allocation statistic
4. **Departmentally Budgeted Personnel Expense**
   Actual = Total actual weekly salary and wage
   Budget = Total budgeted weekly salary and wage
5. **Purchased Services Supply and Expense**
   Actual expense for items/service used by the unit or individuals (e.g., phone, supplies, repairs)
6. **Total Departmentally Budgeted Expense**
   Actual = Personnel expense + nonpersonnel expense
   Budget = Budgeted expense + budgeted nonpersonnel expense
7. **Allocated Departmental Expense**
   Using an allocation statistic (e.g., percentage square feet occupied multipled by dollar amount), a portion of the expense for each department directly related to the unit is calculated and expensed to that cost center
8. **Overhead Expense**
   Using an allocation statistic, a portion of the expense for cost determined to be overhead is expensed to the cost center
9. **Total Revenue**
   Treatment charges generated by the cost center

tion delays, severity of patient/client illness, and therapist's illness. A common unit of measurement is a 60% productivity rate or 20 units of treatment per day per staff therapist. A senior therapist's rate is adjusted for supervisory and teaching responsibilities, for example, a therapist responsible for ward rounds might only be expected to complete 16 units per day allowing 1 hour for rounds.

Each therapist (full-time equivalent, or FTE) is scheduled to work a 40-hour week Monday through Friday, unless assigned to work the weekend. For each day worked a therapist receives a half hour break and a half hour lunch. Thus, they are on-site for 8.5 hours, paid for 8 hours, and available 7.5 hours for assigned duties. Approximately 5 hours (60%) of a therapist's day is expected to be in direct patient care (chargeable) activities.

All direct patient care, note writing and chart review, portal to portal charge for home visits, and family conferences are included in the treatment unit charge. Nonchargeable time includes rounds, team conferences, set-up time, professional consultation, meetings, teaching, student supervision, and educational activities.

An example of a productivity report is seen in Table 4-6. The report presents allocated staff, present staff, and treatment units generated weekly for OT on the inpatient section of the department.

Staff allocated (see Table 4-6, Columns 3, 5, and 8) represents the number of FTE positions budgeted for OT inpatients, which includes all productive and nonproductive hours. The number of staff present (see Table 4-6, Columns 6 and 9) represents only productive hours excluding supervisory overhead and nonproductive hours (vacation, sick, and holiday time). In this example, weekend productivity is considered separately. Most therapists find that they are able to attain a higher rate on weekends as interruptions and delays are minimal, as is nonchargeable time.

Table 4-5
Outpatient Occupational Therapy Service Charge

Provider:	**Date of Visit:**
Diagnosis:	**Date of Onset:**
ICD9 Code:	**Outpatient OT:**

OT	# Units
OT Evaluation	
OT Treatment	
Back School	
UE Physical Cap Eval	
OT Modality	
OT Work Modality	
Therapeutic Pool	
Adaptive Equipment I	
Adaptive Equipment II	
Splint Category I	
Splint Category II	
Splint Category III	
Splint Category IV	
Splint Category V	
Splint Category VI	
Splint Category VII	

The personnel budget of staff salaries and benefits account for approximately 80% of the costs. It reflects all paid hours for staff including regular time, holiday time, weekend differential, overtime, and benefit time scheduled and unscheduled. The latter can be referred to as nonproductive time (i.e., vacation or sick time, professional/conference time, etc.). The statistic gives a true indication of the number of hours worked and the cost of each person in the area.

The nonpersonnel budget addresses the supplies and expenses needed to run the department. For example, it can include office supplies, telephone, lab coats, beepers, travel and education expenses, and splinting and adaptive equipment supplies. Other nonpersonnel considerations are employee benefit expenses, institutional overhead, and allocated costs.

Revenue is the amount of fiscal reimbursement an institution can expect. It is usually based on the charges that the department generates. A cost accounting system determines revenue projections (Macleod, 1971; Mistarz, 1984). This system defines the units of service produced by each ancillary department, such as OT. It provides reports that enable department managers to monitor the variable cost of each unit of service over time and the full cost of ancillary services to determine whether the cost of patient care will exceed per case reimbursement. Such a management reporting system is one based on RVUs (Logigian & Trisolini, 1987). This system is both useful for management and practical to develop.

A RVU system is developed in five steps. The first step is to define outputs. An output is the service or type of therapy provided. Outputs are defined by identifying the variable costs for each service provided. Variable costs are those with no fixed value (i.e., the costs are changeable). To do

Table 4-6
Monthly Productivity Report

Month: February
Section: Inpatient
Therapists: OT

Weekdays

(1) Week Begin	(2) Week End	(3) # FTEs Allocated Per Day	(4) # Days in Week	(5) # FTEs Allocated Per Week (3x4)	(6) # Staff Present in Week	(7) # Time-Based Units in Week	(8) # Units Per FTE Allocated (7/5)	(9) # Units Per Staff Present (7/6)
1	5	5	5	25	17.3	350	14.0	20.29
8	12	5	5	25	20.8	432	17.3	20.77
16	19	5	4	20	16.3	338	16.9	20.74
22	26	5	5	25	17.4	370	14.8	21.26
29	3/4	5	1	5	3.0	68	13.6	22.67

Weekends

(1) Sat.	(2) Sun.	Holiday	(3) # FTEs Allocated Per Day	(4) # Days in Week	(5) # FTEs Allocated Per Week (3x4)	(6) # Staff Present in Week	(7) # Time-Based Units in Week	(8) # Units Per FTE Allocated (7/5)	(9) # Units Per Staff Present (7/6)
6	7	15	1	2	2	2	24	22.50	22.50
13	14		1	3	3	3	72	24.00	24.00
20	21		1	2	2	2	43	21.50	21.50
27	28		1	2	2	2	41	20.50	20.50

Courtesy of the Department of Rehabilitation Services, Brigham and Women's Hospital, Boston, MA.

this, revenue charge codes used by a department can be summarized into categories containing charge items with similar variable costs. For example, all OT 15-minute time charges are grouped into one category since they have the same variable cost. A therapist can provide range of motion, therapeutic exercise, and homemaking activities during a 1-hour treatment session. The category would be called "Occupational Therapy—15 minutes" and the charge would be 4 units. Tables 4-7 and 4-8 give examples of output definitions. Table 4-8 streamlines the process by consolidating outputs.

The second step is to identify the unit cost standards for each output category. Because an OT department budget consists primarily of salaries (80%), it is recommended that all department costs be treated as variable. Fixed costs are those that are not variable (i.e., the costs are not changeable). Equipment and overhead which are considered fixed costs can be captured in separate, indirect cost centers by the institution. Since output categories are defined as groups of charge items with similar costs, unit costs can be developed for each of the output categories. Expected labor and supply costs are calculated and added to find the total expected per unit variable cost for each category. For example, Table 4-9 displays examples of the results of these calculations for the output categories OT, OT modality, and a wrist splint. Similar estimated costs are developed for all output categories listed in Table 4-9, Column 2.

Table 4-7
Examples of Traditional Occupational Therapy Outputs

- OT Evaluation
- Hand Evaluation
- Therapeutic Exercise
- Perceptual Motor Training
- ADL Training
- Dexterity Exercises
- Joint Protection
- Fluidotherapy
- Ultrasound
- Neck Splint
- Wrist Splint
- Hand Resting Splint
- Finger Splint
- CMC Splint

Table 4-8
Examples of Streamlined Occupational Therapy Outputs

- OT—15 Minutes
- OT Modality
- Splint Category I ($0 to $25 cost of materials)
- Splint Category II ($26 to $50 cost of materials)
- Splint Category III ($51 to $75 cost of materials)

Table 4-9
Identifying Variable Costs for Each Output Category

Charge Code/ Output	(1) Time	(2) Average Wage (Salary + 24% Fringe)	(3) Total Time Cost (1x2)	(4) Materials Costs	(5) Total Variable Cost (3+4)
OT	15 minutes	$0.41/minute	$ 6.20	$ 0.00	$ 6.20
OT Modality	60 minutes	$0.41/minute	$24.60	$ 7.58	$32.18
Splint Category II (*wrist splint)	0 minutes	$0.41/minute	$ 0.00	$23.76	$23.76

*Splint fabrication time is included in "OT" time unit charge.

Calculating Variable Cost of Each Charge Code

Splint	(1) Splinting Material	(2) Splinting Material Cost	(3) Velcro Cost	(4) Total Material Cost (2+3)
Wrist Splint	Orthoplast	$20.40	$3.36	$23.76

Table 4-10
Calculating RVUs Using Variable Costs

(1) Charges Codes: Treatment	(2) Variable Cost Per Charge Code	(3) RVUs per Charge Codes (2) 46.20
101: OT—15 Minutes	$ 6.20	1.0
102: OT Modality	$ 32.18	5.2
103: Splint Category I	$ 7.78	1.3
104: Splint Category II	$ 23.76	3.8
105: Splint Category III	$ 39.75	6.4
106: Splint Category IV	$ 55.73	9.0
107: Splint Category V	$ 71.28	11.5
108: Splint Category VI	$119.23	19.2
109: Splint Category VII	$190.51	30.7

Table 4-11
RVU Report for April, Department of Rehabilitation Services
(Cost Center: Inpatient Therapy)

Cost Center Output Categories	(1) Actual April Unit Volume	(2) Budgeted Monthly Unit Volume	(3) Per Unit RVUs	(4) Total Actual RVUs (1x3)	(5) Budgeted RVUs (2x3)
OT	1,521	1,500	1.0	1,521.0	1,500.0
OT Modality	7	5	5.2	36.4	26.0
Splint Category I	2	1	1.3	2.6	1.3
Splint Category II	3	2	3.8	11.4	7.6
Splint Category III	4	1	6.4	25.6	6.4
Splint Category IV	3	3	9.0	27.0	27.0
Splint Category V	2	1	11.5	23.0	11.5
Splint Category VI	2	1	19.2	38.4	19.2
Splint Category VII	2	1	30.7	61.4	30.7
Cost Center Total RVUs				**1,746.8**	**1,629.7**

The third step is to calculate RVUs using the per unit variable cost estimates. The unit cost for OT (Table 4-10) is designated to equal 1.0 RVU. The unit costs of all other categories are divided by the unit cost for OT to arrive at the RVU value for each of the other output categories. The complete list of per unit RVUs is displayed in Column 3 of Table 4-10.

Once RVUs are calculated for each output category, a common unit of measure is available for all different services provided by the department. This enables the fourth step of developing a management report to track unit costs over time. Ratios are constructed to find the actual variable cost per RVU for the department. These ratios are then compared with the budgeted, year-to-date, and previous months' variable costs per RVU.

An example of management reports can be seen in Tables 4-11 through 4-13. The first report (see Table 4-11) calculates the total RVUs for each charge code given the unit volume inputs. In this example, the volume of OT services are above budgeted levels for the current month. This resulted in the total RVUs being above budgeted level. This situation could develop due to an increase in patient census that can increase demand for OT services, or productivity could be high with more patients seen and no patients awaiting services.

Table 4-12
Variable Cost Per RVU Report: Flexible Budget Analysis for April
(Cost Center: Inpatient Occupational Therapy)

(1) Total RVUs	(2) Variable Costs*	(3) Variable Cost Per RVU (2/1)	(4) Budgeted RVUs	(5) Budgeted Variable Costs	(6) Budgeted Variable Cost Per RVU (5/4)
1,747	$7,887	$4.51	1,630	$7,700	$4.72

**Variable costs are determined from monthly department budget reports which indicate salaries and expenses for the month.*

Table 4-13
Trend Report: Variable Cost Per RVU
(Cost Center: Inpatient Occupational Therapy)

(1) Budgeted	(2) YTDA*	(3) February	(4) March	(5) April	(6) May
$4.72	$4.68	$4.75	$4.80	$4.51	

**YTDA = year to date average.*

Table 4-12 calculates the variable cost per RVU and compares the current month's figure with the budgeted figure. In this example, variable costs increased very slightly over budget, and the total RVUs are above budgeted levels. This caused the actual variable cost per RVU to fall below the budget level that is a favorable occurrence.

Table 4-13 provides a trend analysis of unit costs. Actual cost per RVU figures for each month are compared with the budgeted and year-to-date average levels. In this example, it is found that unit costs above the budgeted level in February and March dropped below budgeted level in April.

The fifth step is the development of transfer prices which represent the total (variable plus fixed) cost of each type of service. Total costs are needed as they are used to calculate the cost-per-case for analysis of DRGs. As variable costs have been calculated for each charge code, fixed costs must be determined. To find fixed costs, cost reports and cost allocation statistics are studied to estimate the fraction of hospital-wide indirect overhead costs which should be assigned to an OT department, using a refined step-down methodology (Poulsen, 1984). Once total fixed costs are identified, this figure is divided by the budgeted total RVUs to find the budgeted fixed cost per RVU (Table 4-14, Column 4). The fixed cost of each type of therapy was found by multiplying the budgeted indirect cost per RVU by the total RVUs assigned to each charge code. The variable and fixed costs are then added for each charge code to find the total cost used as the transfer price (see Table 4-14, Column 5).

Figures in Table 4-14 range from $9.35 to $287.22, but the absolute dollar amount is not important. OT at $9.35 is provided to patients much more often than a splint in category VII at $287.22. The important point is that the costs transferred to the cost-per-case analyses represent all hospital-related costs of providing OT to patients.

One recurring issue in designing cost accounting systems is distinguishing fixed from variable costs. This system is a straightforward breakdown: labor and supplies are deemed variable, and

Table 4-14
Transfer Prices for Rehabilitation Services

(1) Output Categories	(2) Per Unit RVUs	(3) Variable Costs (2) x $6.20*	(4) Fixed Cost $3.15**	(5) Transfer Price (3)+(4)
OT	1.0	$ 6.20	$ 3.15	$ 9.35
OT Modality	5.2	$ 32.18	$16.38	$ 48.46
Splint Category I	1.3	$ 7.78	$ 4.10	$ 11.88
Splint Category II	3.8	$ 23.76	$11.97	$ 35.73
Splint Category III	6.4	$ 39.75	$20.16	$ 59.91
Splint Category IV	9.0	$ 55.73	$28.35	$ 84.08
Splint Category V	11.5	$ 71.28	$36.23	$107.51
Splint Category VI	19.2	$119.23	$60.48	$179.71
Splint Category VII	30.7	$190.51	$96.71	$287.22

**Budgeted variable cost per RVU = $6.20.*
***Budgeted fixed cost per RVU = $3.15.*

equipment and overhead are deemed fixed. In some cases, this type of breakdown may seem to create a distortion. Certain types of personnel costs (e.g., supervisors and managers) are usually viewed a semi-fixed costs. But this system encourages managers to critically evaluate the breakdown of their time to encourage them to see more patients. If they see more patients while staff therapists maintain their patient care service levels, the unit cost of care will decrease.

Also, the system is not intended to highlight month-to-month fluctuation since unit costs, which could be affected by changing patient loads, spread over inflexible semi-fixed costs. Rather, it highlights trends in unit costs over 3- or 4-month periods, when unit costs should be controllable even given fluctuations in patient census. This longer term view is intended to encourage cost reduction by attrition instead of layoffs by providing managers several months to adjust to decreasing patient volume.

Management reporting systems implemented in all ancillary departments should be linked to a cost-per-case management system to be most effective in reducing costs. Only with an integrated system are assigned costs under the control of the individuals held accountable for these costs. As PCPs are accountable for the cost implications of inpatient stays and the utilization of ancillaries, department managers are responsible for the unit cost of providing requested services.

Finally, Table 4-15 presents a cost analysis for an upper extremity management program. It lists the components mentioned in this chapter that demonstrate how the fixed and variable costs are developed. Revenue is determined using productivity statistics for each revenue-generating (i.e., billable) area. Net revenue figures are included as part of the analysis as this takes into account a mixed payer group and bad debt (non-collection of monies owed). These numbers are important to financial administrators in determining the feasibility of starting up a new program. The analysis reveals that this proposal should clear $483,791 in gross revenue, which suggests that this should be a successful program.

Table 4-15
Ambulatory Upper Extremity Management Program

Variable Costs		
Personnel	**FTE**	**Cost**
Orthopedic hand surgeon	.2	$ 36,225
Hand fellow	.25	10,608
Neurologist	.1	15,525
Hand therapist	2.0	95,680
Occupational therapist	1.0	40,560
Receptionist	.5	14,127
Fringe (25%)		53,181
Total Personnel		**$265,906**
Supplies		
Office supplies		$ 500
Laundry		2,000
Dressings		2,500
Orthotics		10,000
Splint material		40,000
Rehab supplies		5,000
Total Supplies		**$60,000**
Fixed Costs		
Space—Rent 1000 sq ft ($35/sq ft)		$ 35,000
Phone		1,200
Allocated expense (50% sq ft x $151)		75,091
Overhead expense (10% of variable cost)		32,590
Extra depreciation: New equipment		4,500
Total Costs		**$474,287**
Revenue		
Gross therapy revenue		$ 656,158
Deduction (25%) = Net revenue		406,558
Gross MD revenue		416,000
Deduction (40%) = Net revenue		249,600
Total Net Revenue		**$542,078**
Gross Operating Margin Profit/Loss		**$483,791**
Net Operating Margin Profit/Loss		**$181,871**

Questions

1. To justify the need for more OT aides in a large OT department, you would:
    a. Need to determine current staff productivity
    b. Establish service requirements for all staff
    c. None of the above
    d. Both a and b

2. Which of the following help to decrease length of stay in an acute care hospital?
    a. Establishing a hotel or diagnostic unit adjacent to the hospital
    b. Providing pre-admission and outpatient testing
    c. Providing weekend OT
    d. All of the above

3. Hospital costs have increased because of:
    a. Greater utilization of ancillary services
    b. An increase in government-sponsored health care programs
    c. Salary increases for health care workers
    d. All of the above

4. DRG stands for:
    a. Disability-related group
    b. Diagnosis-related group
    c. Diagnosis-regulated government intervention
    d. None of the above

5. Ways for hospitals to control costs include:
    a. Decreasing length of stay
    b. Increasing productivity
    c. Implementing managed health care plans
    d. All of the above

6. To define outputs, the OT department must:
    a. Summarize into categories charge items with similar variable cost
    b. Only summarize fixed costs
    c. Both a and b
    d. None of the above

7. Which of the following statements is true?
    a. Management reporting systems should be linked to cost-per-case analysis
    b. Productivity should not be linked to cost control strategies
    c. Physicians are the only health care providers who can control costs
    d. OTs have no impact on case mix analysis

8. To limit hospital spending, the federal government:
    a. Increased retrospective payment rates for Medicare recipients
    b. Enacted prospective payment rates for Medicare recipients
    c. Insisted on an increase in length of hospital stay
    d. None of the above

9. Which of the following statements is true?
   a. HMOs have decreased in number throughout the United States
   b. HMOs cannot negotiate rates for per case reimbursement
   c. HMOs have grown significantly in recent years
   d. None of the above

10. PPOs represent:
   a. The greatest growth area in terms of delivery changes
   b. A means of controlling health care costs
   c. Both a and b
   d. None of the above

Case Study 1

The OTs in an acute care teaching hospital want to develop their role in the back school program. Specifically, they want to include a session of work simulation for homemaker back problems. The director of OT agreed that this was an important intervention and asked the therapists to provide a cost analysis of this activity.

The therapists must first define the output that is called work simulation. The variable cost of this service was identified as follows:

Output	Time	Wage	Time Cost	Materials Cost	Total Cost
Work Simulation	45 min	0.41/min	18.45	0.39	$18.84

Materials Analysis	Materials	Cost/Total	Cost/Individual
Work Simulation	Coffee (Can)	5.50	0.05
	Milk (Carton)	0.50	0.05
	Sugar (Packet)	0.05	0.05
	Cups (24 cups)	2.00	0.08
	Snack (12 servings)	2.00	0.16

If the unit cost for OT is equal to 1 RVU as seen in the example in the chapter and 1 RVU is equal to $6.20, the RVU for work simulation is 3.0. Finally, using the formula in the chapter, the transfer price for this output is $18.84 + 3.15 = $21.99.

Case Study 2

The OT department at the Rehabilitation Hospital has recently had an increase in referrals for outpatient therapy. The department head must decide how to handle these referrals. The therapists want the hospital to hire more therapists, but the administration does not want to increase the payroll. The following report is the productivity report for each section of OT for the last 4 weeks. Based on this report, what should the department head recommend?

The report shows that the inpatient therapists were not meeting the productivity level of 22 units per day. As a result, one therapist will be temporarily transferred to the outpatient area to handle the increase in outpatient referrals. If this increase in referrals continues, the department head must carry out a more detailed cost analysis to determine if an additional staff person should be hired.

Case Study 2, Table A

Productivity Report
Month: June
Section: Inpatient
Therapists: OT
Productivity Standard: 22 units (1 unit = 15 minutes)

(1) Week	(2) # FTEs Allocated/ Day	(3) # of Days	(4) # FTEs Allocated (2x3)	(5) Staff Present	(6) Units/Week	(7) Units/FTE Allocated (6-4)	(8) Units/Staff Present (6-5)
4-8	17	5	85	51.0	965	11.4	18.9
11-15	17	5	85	54.5	941	11.1	17.3
18-22	17	5	85	54.0	932	11.0	17.3
25-29	17	5	85	56.8	1027	12.1	18.1

Case Study 2, Table B

Productivity Report
Month: June
Section: Outpatient
Therapists: OT

(1) Week	(2) # FTEs Allocated/ Day	(3) # of Days	(4) # FTEs Allocated (2x3)	(5) Staff Present	(6) Units/Week	(7) Units/FTE Allocated (6-4)	(8) Units/Staff Present (6-5)
4-8	5	5	25	20.0	460	18.4	23.0
11-15	5	5	25	25.0	583	23.3	23.3
18-22	5	5	25	22.5	550	22.0	24.4
25-29	5	5	25	22.5	516	20.1	22.9

References

Coddington, D. C., Palmquist, L. E., & Trollinger, W. V. (1985). Strategies for survival in the hospital industry. *Harvard Business Review, 5*, 129-133.

Evashwick, C. (1989). Creating the continuum of care. *Healthcare Matrix VII, 1*, 30-39.

Goldsmith, J. (1989, May-June). A radical prescription for hospitals. *Harvard Business Review*, 104-111.

Heinemamum, A. W. (1988). Prospective payment for acute care: Impact on rehabilitation hospitals. *Arch Phys Med Rehabil, 69*(8), 614-618.

Lanute, D. (1994). Capitation. *Advance Rehab, 10*, 29-32.

Logigian, M. K. (1987). Productivity analysis. *Am J Occup Ther, 41*(5), 285-291.

Logigian, M. K., & Trisolini, M. G. (1987). A cost analysis and management reporting system in occupational therapy. *Am J Occup Ther, 41*(5), 292-296.

Macleod, R. K. (1971). Program budgeting works in nonprofit institutions. *Harvard Business Review, 9*, 46-56.

Marqulies, N., & Duval, J. (1984, Winter). Productivity management: A model for participative management in health care organizations. *Health Care Management Review, 1*(6), 1-70.

Mistarz, J. E. (1984). Cost accounting: A solution, but a problem. *Hospitals, 9*, 96-101.

Orefice, J. J., & Jennings, M. C. (1984). Productivity—A key to managing cost-per-case. *Health Care Financing Management, 8*, 18-24.

Palmer, B. A. (1996). On managed care. *AOTA Administration Management News, 12*(1), 3-4.

Poulsen, G. P. (1984). Detailed costing system nets efficiency savings. *Hospitals, 10*, 106-111.

Shields, M. D., & Young, S. M. (1992, Spring). Effective long-term cost reduction: A strategic perspective. *Journal of Cost Management, Manufacturing, and Industry,* 16-30.

The preferred provider organization: A response to the environment. (1984, Winter). *Topics in Health Care Financing.*

Vasquez, B. J. (1996). Downsizing: Its effects on clinical staff members. *AOTA Administration Management News, 12*(1), 1-2.

Viewpoints. (1996, February 19). *OT Week,* 46.

Vladeck, B. C. (1984). Medicare hospital payment by diagnosis related groups. *Ann Intern Med, 100,* 576-591.

Woolhandler, S., & Himmelstein, D. U. (1989). Resolving the cost/access conflict: The case for a national health program. *J Gen Intern Med, 4,* 54-60.

Suggested Readings

Bell, N. (1994). The trend towards capitation: The basis for the movement. *Medical Interface, 7*(12), 56-60.

Bray, N., Carter, C., Dobson, A., Watt, J. M., & Shortell, S. (1994). An examination of winners and losers under Medicare's prospective payment system. *Health Care Manage Rev, 19*(1), 44-45.

Carroll, D. (1995). Talking heads: Lesson on capitation. *Trustee, 48*(2), 28.

Cleverly, W. O. (1995). Understanding your hospital's true financial position and changing it. *Health Care Manage Rev, 20*(2), 62-73.

Coile, R. C. (1994). Eight strategies for capitation. *Hospital Strategy, 6*(12), 4-8.

Eckholm, E.(1995). How capitation is transforming hospitals and their staffs. *Med Econ, 72*(10), 45-47.

Finkler, S. A. (1995). Capitated hospital contracts: The empty beds versus filled beds controversy. *Health Care Manage Rev, 20*(3), 88-91.

Fritz, L. R., & Vonderfecht, D. (1994). Radical cost cutting. *Hospital Healthcare Network, 68*(24), 68.

Fritz, L. R., & Wagner, J. (1995). Finding your way through the hospital cost-reduction maze. *Strateg Healthc Excell, 8*(2), 9-12.

Fusco, R. (1994). Home care. An emerging solution to the healthcare crisis. *Hospital Topics, 72*(4), 32-34.

Health maintenance organizations gain popularity, increase capitation. (1995). *OR Manager, 11*(6), 27.

Hirsch, G. B., & Kemeny, J. M. (1994). Mastering the transition to capitation. *Healthcare Forum Journal, 37*(3), 89-91.

Kertesz, L. (1995). Managed-care contracts up, but capitation hits just 40% of California providers-study. *Mod Healthc, 25*(17), 28.

Kolb, D. S. (1995). Managing the transition to capitation. *Healthc Financ Manage, 49*(2), 64-69.

Lumsdon, K. (1994). Ready for cost cutting? One hospital mobilizes its resources. *Hosp Health Netw, 68*(23), 62.

Managed care. (1992). *Hospitals, 66*(17), 17-18.

McCann, K. (1998). HCFA proposes sweeping changes. *OT Week, 7*(9), 12-14.

Miller, T. R. (1995). Managed care. The case for case-based pricing. *Healthc Financ Manage, 49*(7), 22-23.

Rondinelli, R. D., Murphy, J. R., Wilson, D. H., & Miller, C. C. (1991). Predictors of functional outcome and resource utilization in inpatient rehabilitation. *Arch Phys Med Rehabil, 72*(7), 447-453.

Rosenstein, A. H. (1994). Cost-effective health care: Tools for improvement. *Health Care Manage Rev, 19*(2), 53-61.

Sarafini, M. W. (1995). Medicrunch. *National Journal: Washington, 27*(30), 1036-1039.

Sumner, A. T., & Moreland, C. C. (1995). The potential impact of diagnosis related group medical management on hospital utilization and profitability. *Health Care Manage Rev, 20*(2), 92-100.

Toso, M. E., & Farmer, A. (1994). Using cost accounting data to develop capitation rates. *Hospital Cost Management and Accounting, 6*(1), 1-8.

Answer Key

1. d
2. d
3. d
4. b
5. d
6. a
7. a
8. b
9. c
10. c

CHAPTER 5

Supervision

Nancy MacRae, MS, OTR/L, FAOTA

Supervision is a complex and dynamic concept that is inherent in our socialization as professionals. It is a necessary vehicle for facilitating and assessing skill development as beginning practitioners and for ongoing feedback as experienced ones. It is a process which promotes, establishes, maintains, and elevates a level of performance and service (*Guide for Supervision of Occupational Therapy Personnel*, 1994). This definition implies that it is dynamic and reciprocal as well as a collaborative learning relationship for all involved. This view is inherently positive and sets a tone for growth and mutuality. Individuals who enter a supervisory partnership with these assumptions are likely to find the experience rewarding.

Supervision is an important underpinning for our profession's ever-evolving foundation of skills. Supervisors help shape clinical practice. They are necessary for beginning professionals for modeling, support, and assurance of strengthening and refining skill development. Although as a professional matures, the reasons and expectations for supervision change, yet the need for a relationship fostering mutual growth remains. Viewed in this manner, it can remain a vital part of lifelong learning within the profession.

Supervision is a multi-faceted concept that should utilize a systems approach. It occurs in context of an organization, requiring a thorough understanding of it to be effective. Its organizational parameters influence how communication and authority are channeled and, therefore, how tasks are assigned and implemented.

Supervisors are seen as middle managers and are the connecting link between the administration and staff (Haimann, 1989; Umiker, 1988). Administration represents the executive branch of an organization. Its charge is to set policy and provide direction for the organization. Management's role is to direct and maintain the day-to-day operations. It implements policy and as such needs to identify resources and find ways to accomplish the goals of the organization.

Managers are often responsible for one or more units or departments. Supervisors directly oversee the staff who provide the services to meet the goals of the organization. Adding to the complexity is that a person can have administrative, management, and supervisory tasks in one position.

A supervisor's job requires flexibility and the ability to balance component parts to fit the needs. As a leader the supervisor guides others. For others to want to follow, the supervisor needs to possess the powers of persuasion and instill a sense of trust.

Leadership

The leadership aspect of supervision is based on modeling which is characterized by the ability to represent, reconcile, structure, encourage and enhance participation, reward, persuade, predict, and problem solve. Staff are influenced by supervisors who are considerate and capable. Those who have well-performing staff see themselves as effective, tolerant, and have a participatory management style (Brollier, 1985).

Emphasis should be placed on the ability of the supervisor to coach and enable staff to do their jobs. Coaches listen, set limits, shape values such as integrity and trust, and challenge (i.e., encourage skill building). They are task masters yet participate, are accessible, highly visible, provide support, and advocate for staff (Peters & Austin, 1985).

How a supervisor views this role will affect performance style. If it is assumed that people dislike work and try to avoid it, the supervisor may utilize tight control, favor centralized authority, and exhibit authoritarian practices where subordinates' participation is discouraged. In contrast to this view is the assumption that work is as natural to people as play and rest. People will not avoid it. They are self-motivated, gain an inherent satisfaction from work, are committed and motivated, and may seek more responsibility. Those who follow this view utilize a decentralization of authority, democratic practices, and encourage participation of those supervised (Haimann, 1989).

Another conceptual model built on the above is referred to as Theory Z (Ouchi, 1981). It assumes that workers have good ideas and are motivated. Leaders who ascribe to this create trust and open communication by providing a stable environment with a well-articulated philosophy. They provide job enrichment by rotation, de-emphasize hierarchy, delineate career paths, and promote decisions by consensus. In addition, participative decision making is encouraged through the use of quality circles. These are groups of workers from all levels who meet routinely to identify and solve organizational problems (Johnson & Stinson, 1978).

An alternative model for leadership is known as servant leadership (Greenleaf, 1977). Its principles are worth considering in reviewing the process of supervision. Servant leaders put the power in the hands of those they are leading (Dykstra, 1995). Transformative leadership empowers others by committing people to action and converting followers into leaders and leaders into agents of change (Gilfoyle, 1987a). Helping those you supervise to realize they have the power to determine their own professional future is akin to facilitating clients. This type of leadership speaks to the leader's ability to expect growth in supervisees and facilitate it. With such expectations proffered in a fertile milieu, supervisees can experience a surge in their clinical and professional skills. Reinforced training can lead to a desire to grow. Realizing your supervisory style and leadership has enhanced professional growth in those you have supervised can bring with it significant job satisfaction for the supervisor.

Successful supervisors are able to maintain productive relationships through active listening, using such techniques as reflection and introspection, and through learning from their mistakes. They are proactive and able to prioritize and energize others. They are able to integrate vision and values with purpose and promote systems thinking. They teach others to understand the increasing complexity in organizations and assist in building a broad consensus. In addition, they remain sensitive to the supervisee (*Quality Plus II*, 1994).

Successful supervision can be characterized as validation, promptness in responding to a request or need, follow-up on specific issues, and consistency. The abilities to listen, laugh, and motivate staff are important. To be patient and accept the notion that there is more than one way to solve a problem or perform a job are additional attributes of a successful supervisor. Cooperative resolution of problems, often involving creativity and brainstorming techniques, with an inherent trust and respect of each other, are also useful. The ability to model acceptable behavior and appropriate techniques is valuable and may be more meaningful than words to supervisees. The ability to be decisive and act, garnering input from appropriate staff prior to decision making, helps, as is working within the system and utilizing established and accepted practices of communication.

Supervisory Competencies

The ability to enable, educate, and administer are seen as crucial for supervisory success (Gilfoyle, 1987b). Interpersonal relationships permeate the act of supervising and often account for its success in them or a demise. Supervision can make a significant difference in a supervisee's ability to work productively. Access to advice, consultation, and direction is particularly important during times of uncertainty or crisis.

Effective supervisors enjoy people, possess interpersonal skills, and consistently demonstrate care for those with whom they work. This approach leads to a caring management style, which is achieved by setting clear, precise, performance standards and modeling what is desired. Modeling is the most powerful and personal teaching tool available. Self-esteem, self-knowledge, and caring for oneself are prerequisites in effective supervision. An important part of self-knowledge is identifying your own style of supervision. Many different styles have been identified but most can be classified into one of the following four types:

1. **Autocratic.** One person leadership where discipline reigns and staff are seen as cogs in the machine.
2. **Custodial.** Emotional support is blended with authority, leading to a comfortable environment where staff are happy.
3. **Supportive.** Group leadership with staff input and multidirectional communication.
4. **Collegial.** Mutual contribution and commitment to task achievement are evident, and staff are self-motivated and exhibit a high sense of responsibility.

Knowing in which style you are most comfortable, but realizing that your approach may be dictated by the specific situation, can increase your ability to deal promptly, efficiently, and effectively with daily happenings.

As important as identifying your own style is the understanding of the developmental level, personality, and approach of each staff member. In order to enable those you supervise, each staff needs to be seen as an individual, with a unique world perspective. This is imperative with students and new graduates as no assumptions about their knowledge base can be made. Perry's (1968) work on the developmental levels of thinking, or the ability to make your own meaning, can be a helpful framework. Making meaning can be simplified into four levels:

1. Dualism
2. Multiplicity
3. Contextual relativism
4. Commitment within relativism

Explanations of the first three levels, the tasks and challenges involved, and the potential role of both the supervisor and peers are included in Table 5-1.

The supervisor can serve as a bridge linking the old with the new validating a dialectic mode of thought. This individual can introduce the entry-level therapist to the parameters of OT, as well as its

Table 5-1
Characteristics Implied by Perry's Schema

	Dualism	Multiplicity	Contextual Relativism
View of Knowledge	(Conscientious) right and wrong	(Explorer) some certainty remains, most uncertain	(Achiever) all knowledge contextual (rules of adequacy)
Role of Supervisor	Source of knowledge	May discount, as beginning to think about process of thinking	Source of expertise, mutual learning authority via expertise
Role of Student/ Beginning Therapist	Learn right answers, perform right treatment	Learn to think (support with evidence)	"Meta thinking,"use thinking in various contexts
Peer Role in Learning Process	Not a legitimate source of knowledge	A legitimate source of knowledge	Seek out diversity of opinions and expertise, process important
Evaluation Issues	Evaluation clearcut	Value independent thought, qualitative criteria	Separate from self and opportunity for feedback (process of learning)
Primary Intellectual Tasks	Part of whole	Compare, contrast, analyze—some synthesis	Look for relationships, see complexity and fluidity
Source of Challenge	Uncertainty and ambiguity	Evidence to support opinion, accepting responsibility team	Requirements of choice or commitment
Source of Support	Structure, concrete examples, experiential learning	Diversity, may balk at structure	Diversity, opinions, intellectual mastery, seek help from authority

Adapted from Knefelkamp, L. L., & Comfeld, J. L. (1979, March). *Combining student stages and style in design of learning environment: Using Holland typologies and Perry stages.* Paper presented at American College Personnel Association, Los Angeles, CA.

unresolved dilemmas. This last point is particularly relevant as an acceptance of ambiguity, and uncertainty can help a new therapist deal with the stress of being placed within the fast pace that our health care system currently demands or in the role of the expert professional. An open, honest admission of not knowing the answer, but being willing to find it, can be a freeing experience. This requires timing and careful attention to the new therapist's way of making meaning.

Motivation

Motivating staff to effectively perform their jobs is a major objective of supervision. The challenge is to elicit consistent and sustained job performance from each employee. A helpful distinction is discerning the difference between power, the ability to change someone else's behavior as you desire, and motivation, the ability to change someone's behavior as they desire. The judicious use of power complements a frequently utilized reward system (French, 1985). This view of power and the choice process involved facilitates an understanding of both knowing your staff and their needs for rewards, either tangible or intangible. The challenge is to match staff motivation with an effective reward. Short-term, intangible rewards pay off. Management has the most control over this kind of reward, which remarkably enough, need not cost anything. The only cost is in terms of the energy and foresight involved in recognizing the correct time and then in doing it—actually seeing staff doing the right thing and then saying "good job."

When a supervisor knows the supervisees and has established a frequent method of communication with them, the supervisor should be able to discern any symptoms or unease (boredom with responsibilities, decreased challenge in position) being experienced. In an effort to prevent burnout or losing an employee to another position, it is important to have a frank discussion about the particular dimensions of the job in question and identify what is the source of a problem and what are areas that are not problematic. Further exploration is then needed to focus on what can be changed to help relieve the situation and reinvigorate the "soul" of the staff. It may be that the staff need a change of venue within the institution or new responsibilities, such as supervising students, pursuing a research project, or more flexible work hours that will ease the situation. Whatever it may be, it is then a collaborative effort to determine how the targeted changes can occur and plan how time will be derived to accomplish them.

Education

Knowledge and application of adult education principles can enhance supervisory effectiveness. Androgogical assumptions describe the learner as self-directed, entering the educational activity with richer layers of experience. This individual is ready to learn because of a need to know, often associated with a life task or problem, and having potent internal motivators (Knowles & Associates, 1985). Knowing this, effective supervisors, managers, and administrators need to possess the following characteristics:

- A genuine respect for adults to be self-directing
- The ability to derive satisfaction from accomplishments of others
- The ability to value the experience of others
- A willingness to take risks
- A deep commitment to and skill in involving staff in the organization and educational process
- A deep faith in the potency of the educational process
- The ability to establish warm, empathic relationships
- A commitment to lifelong learning for oneself (Knowles, 1980)

In building a working relationship with staff, a supervisor needs to develop a climate that is conducive to learning. Such a climate includes a spirit of collaboration, mutual trust, support, openness, authenticity, pleasure, and humaneness. Clear expectations of work performance need to be established with those involved in planning and designing their objectives and evaluating their success (Knowles, 1980).

Learning Contracts

Supervision of students has brought to light the need for identifying individual outcomes for learning activities which in turn has led to the utilization of learning contracts. They have been utilized in adult learning and can be effectively applied to therapist supervision, particularly for the entry-level practitioner. It is an agreement that establishes roles, responsibilities, and rights of those involved in the transaction (Opacich & Walens, 1991). The learner assumes responsibility for learning and the supervisor for facilitating the process. A set of learning objectives are established by the supervisor in collaboration with the supervisee. They are appropriate for the specific setting and consistent with the experience level of the supervisee. Together they determine how these objectives will be accomplished and measured within a specific time frame. Differences are discussed and resolved until the contract is mutually agreeable. At this point it is signed by each person involved. Examples of learning contract objectives are: effective documentation skills, effective use and interpretation of standardized assessment tools, and appropriate client/therapist interactions. Figure 5-1 presents a sample learning contract.

Administrative Skills

Administrative aspects of the supervisor's job are ensuring that the mission of the institution is followed and that there is compliance with policies and procedures. The line of accountability follows the chain of command, with the supervisor directly responsible for supervisees. Critical with compliance of these responsibilities, supervisors need to be able to delegate, evaluate, and have effective time management.

Delegation

Delegation makes sense as it can be an important tool in teaching and helping to build self-confidence in staff. Clinical knowledge and experience allow the supervisor to assess what needs to be done, gauge an appropriate schedule, and develop the best ways to accomplish the tasks. The ability to know the strengths and weaknesses of staff allow matching qualities with requirements of the job. However, delegating a task is not the end of the supervisor's responsibility. It is necessary to provide staff with the requisite skills for successfully completing the task. Providing the staff with a certain amount of latitude, coupled with clear expectations, frees the staff to complete the task in their own way. Accepting that there is more than one way to do a job and trusting that the job will be completed can be difficult, particularly for the independent supervisor. Coordinating the provision of therapy, ensuring adequate documentation, providing ongoing continuing education, facilitating interdisciplinary collaboration, and dealing with administrative mandates requires each supervisor to be flexible and quick to prioritize and re-prioritize. These latter skills have assumed critical importance with the rapid changes in health care.

Evaluation

An appraisal of a supervisee's job performance is achieved more effectively when supervision is an ongoing process. Face-to-face supervision that is structured, regular, consistent, and process-oriented helps to establish a solid basis for the exchange of information and timely problem solving. For any feedback to be meaningful, it needs to be supported by appropriate modeling.

Annual and objective appraisals of staff performance by the supervisor are expected to be completed in a thorough and timely manner. Performance appraisals are a formal system of measuring and evaluating employee's job-related activities. They audit the effectiveness of an employee's performance. They need to be based on specific, realistic, and achievable criteria that directly relate to the duties described in the job description. A simple way to remember what needs to be included in a performance appraisal is revealed by using the acronym (Umiker, 1988):

R—Review and clarify expectations
E—Evaluate performance
E—Express appreciation
F—Future planning

Completing a mutually satisfying annual appraisal can be accomplished if there is an established supervisory relationship. If communication about job performance has occurred regularly

Learning contract for:

Objectives	Potential Resource and Strategies	Outcomes	Status	Comments
1. To exercise safety precautions	• Reads relevant policies and procedures • Reviews handling and safety precautions taught at school • Observes therapist's practice of safety procedures • Practices safety procedures with supervision	1. Demonstrates proper body mechanics when handling clients 2. Consistently demonstrates safety precautions in all aspects of client care (transfers) 3. Consistently follows facility's procedures for safety (universal precautions, infection control) 4. Monitors client's medical status to ensure safe treatment—seeks advice when situation deemed unsafe		
2. To demonstrate verbal communication skills	• Contributes in team meetings • Speaks to clients, families, other professionals, and supervisor	1. Verbally contributes clear, concise, and appropriate information on assigned clients in team meetings 2. Demonstrates effective communication with supervisors as issues arise through giving and receiving verbal feedback 3. Clearly conveys OT role through interactions with clients, families, and other professionals 4. Consistently provides clear instructions and demonstration to clients, appropriate for their level of understanding		

Date of Agreement: **Date of Completion:**

Student Signature: **Student Signature:**

Supervisor Signature: **Supervisor Signature:**

Figure 5-1. OT department learning contract.

during the designated time period, the annual appraisal can be a capstone of the year's results. Such an evaluation will hold no surprises and new objectives for the upcoming year will not be difficult to determine. Should the opposite be the case, the meeting may well be fraught with anxiety that will diminish the opportunity for it to be a productive experience.

During the first year of employment, a new staff person is usually evaluated after 3 months, often considered a probationary period, to determine if job performance is consistent with the tasks described in the relevant job description. Level of competency with these tasks will be a determining factor in continuing employment. If enough tasks are being performed adequately, employment continues with specific, realistic, and achievable criteria established for improving the level of performance in identified areas. Typically the next review is in another 3 months. Needed support should be identified for achieving any established short-term goals. In other words, responsibility is assigned the supervisee to meet the established criteria and the supervisor to provide the support necessary for the supervisee to achieve them.

A more frequent practice being used by supervisors today is to have the supervisee complete a self-evaluation prior to the date of the annual review. At the annual review, both will then compare their assessments of performance, discussing any discrepancies. For a new therapist and indeed a new employee, this can be a very challenging task due to lack of comparative data and a tenuous level of self-confidence. It does provide helpful feedback to the supervisee regarding over- or underestimation of ability. This can help the supervisee focus while the supervisor can better determine future learning opportunities.

An identification of objectives for the new year should also be individually determined by the supervisor and the supervisee. Once discussed in relation to actual previous performance, mutually determined objectives need to be devised, with particular attention paid to those that energize/inspire/feed the soul of the supervisee.

A variety of appraisal formats exist. Many institutions have standardized formats for use with all employees. When these forms do not provide the feedback needed, they can be supplemented with written synopses of performance. Staff may appreciate this as it adds weight to the perception that they are being viewed as a unique individual.

Evaluation Forms

Appraisal forms are most often behavior-based, covering such areas as the quantity and quality of work, job knowledge, dependability, attitude, supervision required, safety, personal appearance, communication ability, adherence to policies and procedures, judgment, and initiative. The systems used to do this can include any combination of the following formats:

- **Essay.** Written, time consuming, least structured; usually used in combination with a more structured format.
- **Critical incident.** Daily log of specifics, requires objectivity; may increase worker anxiety.
- **Forced distribution ranking.** Rank according to quality of work, may be difficult to justify.
- **Behavior checklists.** Saves time and minimizes bias; usually includes 10 to 20 items.
- **Linear scale.** Likert scale ranking; tendency to rank in mid-range.
- **Management by objectives.** Jointly established objectives with a time frame; can be time consuming.

Figure 5-2 presents an example of a performance appraisal. Another variation is one that ties individual behaviors with organizational values. This type often emphasizes customer satisfaction with core competencies of initiative, adaptability, decision making, and customer service.

A helpful way to remember how to develop ideal performance objectives is portrayed in the following acronym (Umiker, 1988):

R—Relevant to work goals of both employer and employee
U—Understandable, clear, and specific
M—Measurable and quantitative
B—Behavioral, observable change
A—Achievable

Completed annual evaluations form the basis for decision making regarding job responsibilities, promotions, and pay increases. Productive evaluations are continuous, recapitulating previously shared information. They are discussed in detail so that both parties are clear on the expectations with the focus on work performance, not personality, unless it adversely affects performance. Strengths and weaknesses are presented in a fair and balanced way, with areas of growth identified. A summary statement is also included.

Name **Date**

1. How well does employee manage others? 20 possible points

Secures satisfactory production from unit of responsibility under routine or favorable conditions.	Keen judgment and very accurate decisions, usually unit has high productivity.	Occasionally provides leadership and secure minimum production from subordinates.	Does not exercise leadership; results of unit of responsibility are unsatisfactory.	Outstanding leader; constantly produces maximum from unit by motivating subordinates.	Almost always succeeds, even under unusual or difficult circumstances; controls unit of of responsibility effectively.
6 7 8 9 10	15 16 17 18	2 3 4 5	0 1	19 20	11 12 13 14

Remarks:

2. How well does employee utilize resources? 20 possible points

Consistently effective in utilization of materials and manpower; procedures developed go beyond own operation or responsibility.	Ordinarily conserves material and manpower. Implements and maintains routine management procedures for that purpose.	Ineffective in the conservation of materials and economical use of manpower.	Effective in accomplishing savings in material and manpower. Develop improved management procedures for that end as appropriate.	Utilizes material and manpower in a barely satisfactory manner.	Almost always conserves material and manpower, implements and maintains routine manage ment procedures for that purpose.
19 20	6 7 8 9 10	0 1	15 16 17 18	2 3 4 5	11 12 13 14

Remarks:

3. How effective in planning and organizing the workload? 15 possible points

Causes some practical improvements in improving workloads for unit	Plans workloads of subordinates, but judgment is not always good.	Resourceful in practical adaptions, even in unusual circumstances.	Little aptitude or inclination for devising means for accomplishing unit objective.	Able to anticipate critical events and make prior provisions to deal with them.	Seeks guidance on what is expected of unit more than should be necessary. Does little planning for unit.
8 9 10	5 6 7	11 12 13	0 1	14 15	2 3 4

Remarks:

Figure 5-2. Performance appraisal form—supervisory and management group. Courtesy of the State of Maine, Bureau of Human Resources.

Annual evaluations need to be scheduled and private with distractions kept to a minimum. Most annual evaluation sessions also include a request for feedback on the supervisor's performance (Figure 5-3). This feedback can be the basis for a productive discussion on the effectiveness of supervisory style and needed changes.

Appraisals of staff performance need to include direct observation of performance, review of documentation, and verbal reports of clinical activities. Reports from co-workers, clients, and families can be included where appropriate. The most effective process includes self-appraisal, joint problem solving, and mutual determination of annual objectives. The major goal of the supervisor is to make the employee feel like a winner, that is, an appreciated and valued member of the staff. Defensiveness can be minimized when past performance is used as a database for planning future performance.

Annual appraisals are important documentation of an employee's job history. Other documentation that needs to be considered during the year being reviewed are critical incidents, which can be both positive and negative accounts of specific episodes, and generated from inside and outside of the department. Disciplinary actions must be reviewed as part of the process and can include a verbal warning, written warning, and specific disciplinary action. In a unionized workforce or within a large institution, these procedures are spelled out in detail.

Reward systems are usually linked to the appraisal system. Salary adjustments such as merit increases can be offered, as can verbal or written praise. Continuing education can also be viewed as a reward.

The flip side of support is often a more difficult task for the supervisor because it involves dealing with weaknesses. Being able to constructively criticize a staff member can make the difference between being heard or ignored. The former can become an enabling experience where growth alternatives can be discussed, particularly when it is done within a well-established supervisory pattern. Thus, the importance of frequent communication cannot be overstated.

Additional Considerations

Humor can play a great part in our professional lives. OTs are dedicated, serious professionals. The ability to laugh at oneself, as well as admitting when one is wrong, can provide necessary relief and spawn the renewal needed to continue. Modeling appropriate humor, particularly the ability to laugh at yourself, provides staff with permission to do the same. We need to become more aware of those lighter moments and use them effectively. Humor can become a bonding experience for staff members.

Time Management

An additional important aspect of a supervisor's job is effective time management. As demands increase on clinicians, time becomes a premium. Judicious use of it is crucial if all components of a supervisor's job are to be met. For the supervisor there is time devoted to the organization, including staff and the administration and time that is discretionary (Bair & Gray, 1992). Efficient use of both is necessary to be able to do all that is required to keep a department running smoothly. Modeling effective use of time sets a standard for staff and helps to prevent time thefts.

Time thefts by employees include unscheduled absences, tardiness, leaving early, extended breaks, excessive socialization, completion of personal tasks, and daydreaming. Reasons for such thefts include low morale, lack of interest, boredom, and an inability to understand the work. Recognizing this behavior, setting an example of efficient time use, specifying expectations, coun-

Supervisor Name: **Date:**
Employee Name: **Division/Department:**

To Employee: Please check the category that best describes your thoughts about your supervisor's effectiveness in enabling you to best perform your job.
N = Never O = Occasionally U = Usually A = Always N/A = Not Applicable

My Supervisor:	**N**	**O**	**U**	**A**	**N/A**
1. Explains my job expectations to me.					
2. Provides clear direction.					
3. Is helpful at solving work problems.					
4. Gives fair evaluation and criticism.					
5. Is informed of policies and procedures and keeps me informed.					
6. Informs me of specific ways I can improve my work and where my current performance lies in relation to job expectations and goals.					
7. Recognizes and commends effort and achievement.					
8. Gives me support when I need it.					
9. Is open to constructive criticism.					
10. Listens to my opinions and shows respect for my ideas, even when they are not in agreement with the supervisor's.					
11. Is concerned about me as a person and takes my preferences into account when assigning duties.					
12. Advocates for me.					
13. Makes self available.					
14. Follows through with commitments made.					
15. Promotes an atmosphere where I can request information and guidance comfortably.					
16. Helps me fit my work into the broader context of the organization.					
17. Fosters a team attitude among staff.					
18. Projects a positive attitude about staff.					

Employee Comments:

Supervisor Comments:

Employee Signature: **Date:**

Supervisor Signature: **Date:**

Supervisor's Greatest Strengths:

Supervisor's Greatest Weaknesses:

Changes that would help you do your job better:

Figure 5-3. Supervisory feedback. Used with permission from Judith L. Kimball, PhD, OTR/L, FAOTA, Occupational Therapy Department, University of New England, Biddeford, ME.

seling the worst offenders, changing work sites, and providing staff with an effective workload encourage creative solutions and help control time theft behaviors. Of course, reinforcing desired behaviors is the most powerful tool.

Keeping a time log in 15-minute increments to determine how you spend your time can provide a baseline for determining strategies to improve use of time. Utilizing a desk calendar and a weekly and/or monthly planning sheet for scheduling can help impose realistic organizational parameters on your time use, highlighting when specific demands are due. Eliminating unnecessary tasks is a good first step (i.e., distinguishing between what must be done from what should be done). Delegating more tasks not only helps in your use of time but also builds confidence and facilitates skill building in your staff. Teaching subordinates to solve their own problems by insisting they bring potential solutions to you with their problems can help. Coaching them can increase self-confidence and self-reliance. Practice managing by walking around (Umiker, 1988) on a regular basis. It can be a proactive approach by increasing your accessibility and increasing opportunities to discover staff doing wonderful things. Establishing relevant policies and procedures can eliminate repetitive questions. Organizing work in better ways through an effective filing system, baskets to hold incoming and outgoing papers, and a list of prioritized tasks all help with more efficacious time use. Effective communication with use of good listening skills can keep you in tune with what is being said and the emotional content behind it. Finally, avoiding procrastination can save time, as can being sure to block out sufficient time to complete complex tasks.

The supervisor's job is a critical one within our profession. Our entry into the arena of clinical practice occurs only under the auspices of a supervisor. The characteristics of the initial relationship with a supervisor remains with us. We attempt to emulate those traits that helped us grow and gain self-confidence while we avoid those that were not constructive. Combining supervisory knowledge with clinical experience and interpersonal skills provides the framework for an effective supervisory position. Establishing an environment of support, openness, and trust promotes the ability to enable staff to acquire the skills needed to be successful practitioners. Striving to encourage growth and dependence through modeling can lead the therapist to independence and success as a supervisor.

Remember that how you work and interact with others is directly reflected back to you by your staff and should be used as a real guide for your practice of supervision. Because supervision is a complex job, it is a challenge. Yet, to see on a daily basis how your direction and guidance can help shape both individual practitioners and clinical practice is a genuinely rewarding experience. Effective supervision can make a real difference for our profession and thus for the lives of the clients with whom we work.

Questions

1. Enabling, educating, and administering are components of a supervisor's job. Label each sentence as:

   A. Enabling
   B. Educating
   C. Administering function

   a.__ Jane, the supervisor, makes an effort to remember each of her staff's birthdays.
   b.__ Mark, the clinic manager, insists on compliance of the confidentiality policy and procedures.
   c.__ Julie, a Level II student, worked collaboratively with Jim, her supervisor, to devise objectives for her 3-month experience.
   d.__ Sarah, an experienced therapist and long-time employee, was provided with the opportunity to engage in an interdisciplinary research project on traumatic brain injury by her supervisor.
   e.__ Josh is careful to model a balanced approach to his work for his staff. He arrives early, works diligently, and then most often leaves at the end of the regular work day. Additionally, he exercises each day during his lunch break.

2. Charlotte, a beginning therapist, has stated that her preference for supervision is close at first. Once she begins to feel more comfortable she desires weekly meetings only. You feel that she is ready to assume more autonomy; she remains unsure. What can you do to promote the development of more self-confidence? Check all that apply.

   a.__ Insist that you only have time for one meeting a week; specify time and day of week.
   b.__ Relay your belief in her burgeoning abilities.
   c.__ Assure her you are readily accessible.
   d.__ Encourage her to inform you of what transpired during therapy sessions.
   e.__ Suggest supervision meetings three times a week for 2 weeks, twice a week for 1 week, and then once weekly.
   f.__ Pair her up with another student.
   g.__ Have her assume more responsibility with you in the background, gradually fading out your presence.
   h.__ Provide frequent feedback, positive and constructive, about her performance.

3. Despite frequent reminders and encouragement, Jane is not meeting deadlines for her documentation. Although she does have some severely involved clients on her caseload, her workload is compatible with her peers who are meeting documentation deadlines. Identify the appropriate approaches.

   a.__ Dock her pay.
   b.__ Have her come in to discuss why she is unable to meet deadlines; ask what else is going on in her life.
   c.__ Provide her with help to incorporate better time management skills.
   d.__ Review documentation procedures with her.
   e.__ Buddy her with a peer so she can use her as a model.

4. Dr. Green, a conservative physician who strictly follows protocol, has called you to complain of John's performance during team meeting this morning. He has identified his behavior as disrespectful and aggressive. He wants to discuss the matter before tomorrow's team meeting. How should you proceed? Check all that apply.

   a.__ Ask Dr. Green for further clarification of what he means by "disrespectful" and "aggressive."
   b.__ Meet with John to hear his rendition.
   c.__ Ask another team member for his or her view of what transpired.
   d.__ Go prepared to listen to Dr. Green but also to be clear about your staff's right to voice their clinical opinions and recommendations about client treatment.

5. You are a new supervisor who has a staff of six therapists, one of whom is older than you (by 10 years) and has worked at this facility for 5 years. Since your arrival, she has been cold toward you, making it clear in her behavior that she does not see you as a legitimate authority figure. She has been consistently late for work (two to three times a week) and is always tardy to your departmental meetings (by 5 or 10 minutes). How will you handle this situation? Check all that apply.

a.__ Meet with her and verbally reprimand her for her tardiness.
b.__ Call her on her late arrival at staff meetings.
c.__ Counsel her on her behavior, indicating the effect it has on her peers.
d.__ Ask her to explain the reasons for her behavior.
e.__ Once behavior is rectified, try to delegate more responsibility to her, eventually working her into a position of more authority.

6. Tony, an OTR on your staff, has complained to you about what he considers an unfair practice of the organization for which you both work. He has made it clear that he expects you to fix it. What will you do? Choose the best answer.

a.__ Fix it.
b.__ Acknowledge that you've heard him; insist that he come up with a few possible alternatives when you can meet again so you can collaboratively decide on the best approach.
c.__ Have a more experienced staff person deal with it.

7. A local university has called asking for your help in providing a Level I clinical site for two students who were just cancelled from their prearranged sites. Your census is high and staff are working hard to meet their job responsibilities. What will you do? Identify those answers that are most appropriate and assign an order to the sequence in which they should be done.

a.__ Creatively brainstorm with staff.
b.__ Inform staff; let them think about it overnight.
c.__ Deny the request.
d.__ Meet early the next day to discuss whether it is feasible to take two new students.

8. With the recent increased demand for productivity at the clinic, Ellen, an experienced therapist, has been having difficulty meeting deadlines for completing her documentation of client therapy. How should you proceed to handle this?

a.__ Tell her to shape up.
b.__ Make an appointment to talk with her and then ask her what is going on.
c.__ Counsel her on time management techniques.
d.__ Provide training on using computers to complete documentation.

9. George, a new graduate on his first Level II fieldwork, and his supervisor, Rita, need to write a learning contract for his 3-month experience. The site is a community mental health site where the population is composed primarily of drop-ins throughout the day. Develop an appropriate list of objectives based on his experience level and the site.

10. You are the supervisor of a rapidly expanding rehabilitation clinic. Recent plans to add on space to your existing room have added multiple responsibilities to your already busy schedule. Your staff is composed of therapists with 1, 2, and 3 years of responsibility. Areas of responsibility that need to be delegated are listed below. Match those most appropriate to the therapists labeling them 1, 2, or 3 to coincide with their year of clinical experience.

a.__ Supervision of Level I student.
b.__ Provision of educational sessions to Level II students from OT and PT departments.
c.__ Writing departmental annual report.
d.__ OT representative to rehabilitation meetings.
e.__ Ordering of adaptive equipment.
f.__ Presentation on OT to local women's group.

Case Study 1

You are the clinical supervisor in the burn unit of an acute care hospital and Elaine, an OT with approximately 6 months of clinical experience, is going to be assigned to a 3-month rotation on the burn unit under your supervision.

When you meet with Elaine before the rotation begins, you describe the patient population, discuss the role of the various team members, and discuss the role of the OT in the care of the burn patient. She is asked to come to this preliminary meeting prepared to discuss her prior experience on the previous orthopedic rotation, her perceptions of her clinical strengths and areas for growth, her goals for the upcoming rotation, and her learning style. To gather information about her clinical performance, you review the end of rotation evaluation prepared by her prior supervisor. These are some of the things you learn about Elaine as you gather the above information.

a. She is a better visual learner than auditory learner and has difficulty retaining what has been told to her.
b. After being instructed in what to do, she appreciates the opportunity to practice on her own before the supervisor provides feedback regarding her performance.
c. Elaine feels a strength of hers is teaching the families of her patients how to carry through with exercise programs and activities of daily living skills.
d. Prior splinting experience is limited to the fabrication of two thumb splints for a patient with osteoarthritis of the carpometacarpal joints of both hands.
e. Elaine reports that she is not yet comfortable in transferring patients who need moderate or more manual assistance, and is concerned about her safety in these maneuvers, given that she has recovered from a recent back injury.
f. She has a tendency to spend a lot of time speaking to her patients and providing social-emotional support, to the point where little time is spent on therapeutic activities. Short-term goals might, therefore, go unmet.
g. A primary goal of Elaine's is to be able to manage all aspects of a burn patient's care, including initial evaluation, positioning, splinting, range of motion exercises, activities of daily living, patient and family education, collaboration with other members of the team, reporting at daily rounds, and discharge planning.

Given this information, which of the following patients might you choose to assign as her first?

a. A 69-year-old male with a 50% total body surface third degree burn, affecting primarily his lower extremities. Social service expects there will be a problem with the discharge since he does not have a family who can help in his care when he is discharged.
b. A 50-year-old female with a history of alcohol abuse who sustained a burn injury while smoking in bed intoxicated. The burn affects primarily her face, neck, left upper extremity, and upper chest. Her husband is involved in her care.
c. A 40-year-old female who sustained burns of both upper extremities while cooking on a camping trip with her husband.

1. Discuss the reasons for your choice of intial patient assignment.
2. Set competency outcomes for the splinting segment of a burn rotation. The goals should be objective and measurable.
3. Describe the instructional methods you will select and the steps you will take to teach the goals set in Number 2, given Elaine's learning needs.

Case Study 2

Consider the following scenario. The beginning staff therapist is conducting her first family instruction session. The patient is present and the therapist is showing the husband of the patient how to perform a moderate assist stand pivot transfer into the bathtub. The therapist has demonstrated prior to this that she understands the proper technique, however, the technique she demonstrates is somewhat difficult. The family is asking the therapist for clarification. You, as the supervisor, are looking on from a distance.

1. What will you do and what principles guide your choice of action?
2. Will you say anything and why or why not?
3. What will you say if you do choose to give feedback?

Case Studies courtesy of Bette Hoffman Harel, MS, OTR/L.

References

Bair, J., & Gray, M. (1992). *The occupational therapy manager*. Rockville, MD: American Occupational Therapy Association.

Brollier, C. (1985). Occupational therapy management and job performance of staff. *Am J Occup Ther, 39*, 10.

Dykstra, A. (1995). *Outcome management: Achieving outcomes for people with disabilities*. East Dundee, MI: High Tide Press.

French, M. (1985). *Beyond power: On women, men and morals*. New York: Ballantine.

Gilfoyle, E. M. (1987a). Nationally speaking, leadership and management. *Am J Occup Ther, 41*, 5.

Gilfoyle, E. M. (Ed.). (1987b). Training: Occupational therapy educational management in schools. AOTA, Vol. 4, Module 7, Grant #G007801499 Dept. of Education, Office of Special Education and Rehabilitation Services.

Greenleaf, R. K. (1977). *Servant leadership*. Mahwah, NJ: Paulist Press.

Guide for supervision of occupational therapy personnel. (1994). *Am J Occup Ther, 48*, 11.

Haimann, T. (1989). *Supervisory management for healthcare organizations*. St. Louis: Catholic Health Association of the United States.

Johnson, T., & Stinson, J. (1978). *Managing today and tomorrow*. Reading, MA: Addison-Wesley Publishing Co.

Knowles, M. (1980). *The modern practice of adult education*. Chicago: Follett Publishing.

Knowles, M., & Associates. (1985). *Andragogy in action: Applying modern principles of adult learning*. San Francisco: Jossey-Bass Publishers.

Opacich, K., & Walens, D. (1991). *Structuring the learning experience*. Rockville, MD: American Occupational Therapy Association.

Ouchi, W. G. (1981). *Theory Z: How American business can meet the Japanese challenge*. Reading, MA: Addison-Wesley Publishing Co.

Perry, W. G. (1968). *Forms of intellectual and ethical development in the college years: A scheme*. New York: Holt, Rinehart and Winston.

Peters, T. J., & Austin, N. (1985). *A passion for excellence*. New York: Warner Books.

Quality plus II: Putting outcomes into action. (1994). Towson, MD: The Accreditation Council.

Umiker, W. (1988). *Management skills for the new health care supervisor*. Rockville, MD: Aspen Publishers.

Suggested Readings

Kadushin, A. (1974). Supervisor-supervisee: A survey. *Social Work, 19*.

Answer Key

1. aA, bC, cB, dB, eA
2. c, e, h
3. c, d
4. b, d
5. c, d
6. b
7. a, b, d
8. b, c
9. Please develop
10. a1, b2, c3, d1, e1, f2

CHAPTER 6

Managing Our Limited Resource: Practitioners

Thomas F. Fisher, MS, OTR/L, CCM, FAOTA

Introduction

The primary purpose of this chapter is to discuss the issues relative to recruiting and retaining professional staff. With the advent of managed care, there is the potential of moving into an era where services may be provided to consumers by persons with limited educational preparation in the area of rehabilitation (i.e., rehabilitation technician, aide). It will become increasingly important for managers to understand the internal and external systems where they are employed. OT practitioners are OTRs and COTAs; PT practitioners are PTs and PTAs. These health professionals have much to offer health care and rehabilitation. Moving into the 21st century, universities and colleges have seen the growing need for these professionals and have increased their enrollment with existing programs or have initiated programs that did not exist in the past. In 1998, the AOTA reported there were approximately 121 OTR programs, 20 developing OTR programs, 159 COTA programs, and another 22 developing COTA programs (Accreditation Council for Occupational Therapy Education, 1998). It is projected that by the turn of the century the supply will be better than it has been. Regardless, the challenge of a manager continues to be able to recruit and retain those practitioners that are critical for delivering competent and cost-effective services. If the managed care trend encourages organizations to employ less trained and educated personnel to lower costs, the outcomes of such services will be the measurement of the effectiveness of this trend. Managers need to be aware of these issues and plan accordingly.

As the shortage of allied health professionals continues, specifically OT practitioners, organizations are increasing their expenditures for recruitment and retention of these vital human resources. Salaries, benefit packages, sign-on bonuses, tuition assistance, and referral bonuses are a few expenditures. Since many organizations may experience financial problems, it is important for the manager to know which employment factors have the highest influence on the recruitment and retention of allied health professionals in order to plan appropriately.

Mergers, acquisitions, and joint ventures are all trends that have been occurring over the past several years in health care. For example, in 1994, Continental Medical Systems (CMS), Horizons, and Rehab Works were all separate organizations (McDonald, 1996). During 1996, they all became a part of the same organization. Vencor, an organization of approximately 35 acute care respiratory hospitals, acquired Hillhaven Corporation, a 300+ long-term care organization; 55 retail and institutional pharmacies; and 23 retirement homes in 1995 to be one of the largest health care organizations in the United States. All of these organizations are providers of rehabilitation and will continue to need to recruit and retain OT practitioners. As the public awareness increases regarding disabled individuals and their need to be independent, the growth of rehabilitation should continue. Federal and state regulations currently require that certain populations be entitled to therapy services (i.e., children between the ages of 3 to 21 to benefit from their public education). Another trend that will require the skills and knowledge of OT practitioners is the growing number of the elderly who are at risk for disease and illness. With rehabilitation, many times these individuals can continue to live productive lives. For these reasons, the demand for OT practitioners should continue.

It has been reported that the primary employment factors influencing recruitment and retention of allied health professionals is compensation (salaries), range of services, variety of patients, size of department (number of OTRs and COTAs), reputation for high technology and state-of-the-art procedures, job security, benefits, and opportunity to work the shifts and schedules desired. Additional factors influencing recruitment are location of the organization, reputation for quality patient care, and a positive work environment. Factors influencing retention are the opportunities to achieve personal and professional goals in providing high quality health care (professional self-actualization) and amount of paid time off for vacations and holidays. Since many health care organizations are already experiencing financial problems, it is important for not only the OT manager but the organization to know which employment factors have the highest influence on the recruitment and retention of practitioners in order to make the most of the expenditures allocated. Recruitment and retention has been said to form a productive circle. Quality patient care is at the center of the circle and is surrounded by a continuous chain of recruitment and retention (Dawe & Smith, 1988). This analogy suggests that if the chain were to have a break in it, typically the quality of care would be sacrificed. Let us look at each of these issues separately.

Recruitment

Recruitment of health professionals was the main concern of organizations in the 1980s. However, retention has become the emphasis during the 1990s. Recruitment is defined as the action or process of recruiting; the process of adding new individuals to a population or subpopulation by growth (*Webster's Collegiate Dictionary*, 1993). Professional recruiters have become the largest population of exhibitors at the annual AOTA conferences. In 1992, the AOTA reported salaries for OTRs and COTAs had risen by approximately 8% annually since 1986 and by 9% annually for new graduates. Anecdotally, it has been found that a growing number of OT students are securing employment in return for financing their professional education. Other successful recruitment methods are word-of-mouth, newspaper ads, and college placement services. In 1992, it was reported that 90% of placement chairpersons in state OT associations said there were more jobs than personnel for OTs in their states and almost 80% concurred the same problem for OTAs (Silvergleit, 1992). Besides a growth in personnel recruiters, there has also been growth in traveling therapy companies, temporary agencies, and firms that recruit foreign-trained therapists because of this personnel shortage. It has been found that the recruitment process is costly and frustrating for many health care organizations. Using contact therapy is a quick alternative for many organizations. Employers continue to evaluate what both therapists and assistants want in a job. The recruitment process has seven basic steps:

1. Identification of the position
2. Attracting the applicant
3. Screening
4. Interview
5. Checking references
6. Job offer
7. Follow-up

The first step is the identification of the position. This is the clarification of the job duties and essential functions, a job description. Describing the essential job functions and educational requirements would be part of this step. The next step is to attract applicants. This is accomplished in a variety of ways. Advertising in trade journals and state OT newsletters is one frequent method used by employers. Networking both internally (within the organization) and externally (outside the organization) is also recommended. Many times employees from other departments within the organization may know an OT or know someone who knows an OT. Being involved in professional organizations is a method of learning what employees are looking for and which practitioners are considering a change in employment. If a connection happens, this may have occurred without the cost of advertising.

Once a qualified applicant has been identified, the next step is screening applicants for an interview. The manager will typically review the applications and résumés determining who meets the predetermined criteria for the position. Interview dates are then scheduled. The OT manager should be aware of the significant employment legislation when going through this process (i.e., Civil Rights Act of 1964, Titles VI and VII [as amended in 1972], Rehabilitation Act of 1973, Section 504, and the ADA). The interview has become a critical step in the recruitment process. The interview can be formal or informal. The method used should allow the interviewer to obtain the needed information. Obtaining, verifying, and transmitting are skills the OT manager must use during the interview. The structure of the interview should allow for appropriate information to be obtained, career goals and needed skills verified, and a synopsis of the interview transmitted. Written information about the organization and benefits should be given to the interviewee/candidate. During the interview, as many staff and administrative persons as appropriate should meet with the candidate(s). The OT manager can then receive feedback from many different sources in order to make an informed decision. Impressions regarding appearance, poise, interpersonal communication skills, knowledge in the field, and compatibility with the organization are just a few of the areas that staff could assess about the candidate(s). Based on the interviews, typically there is a decision made of which candidate(s) will remain active and those who will be eliminated. All candidates interviewed should be informed when a decision will be made and how they will be contacted.

The next step of the interview process is the checking of references. Unfortunately, most employers only provide the dates an employee was employed. In the past, employers would indicate whether they would rehire the employee. This is no longer common practice. Reference checks are done over the telephone and through the mail. Typically, the reference is over the telephone, because it allows more flexibility. Because of the shortage of OT practitioners, managers sometimes consider skipping this step (Parisi, 1994). It is the ethical responsibility of the manager to secure these references before an offer is extended. This step can be time consuming but it provides the supporting information to the manager about the candidate(s).

The next step in the recruitment process is the job offer. After the references have been received, the manager will make a decision based on the application/résumé information, the interview(s), and the references. The job offer is discussed over the telephone and followed up in writing. The job offer includes salary, terms of employment, and a starting date. If the candidate accepts the offer, the manager should provide the candidate with state licensure information, particularly if the person is coming from out of state.

The final step is follow-up. After the manager has verbally reached an agreement with the candidate, a confirmation letter is sent. This provides written evidence of the terms of the employment as well as follow-up communication. Reminders about where to park, dress code, and a tentative schedule is also suggested. It has also been recommended that if more than 1 month passes from the time of the offer and the start date, a phone call is recommended (Parisi, 1994). Only after this step should the remaining candidates who were interviewed be notified that the position has been filled. The manager should also include a statement of whether they might be considered for future positions (Schell, 1992).

Retention

It is extremely important that OT managers be successful at recruitment. However, during the past several years, retention has surpassed recruitment in importance. Retention is defined as the state of being retained or the act of retaining (*Webster's Collegiate Dictionary*, 1993). The challenge for the OT manager is to understand and accept the needs of the staff. As stated earlier, salaries, benefit package, variety of patients served, reputation for state-of-the-art technology and procedure, and job security are a few of the issues that influence retention (Makely & Bamberg, 1991). Besides these, personal and professional growth and development affect retention. Job satisfaction fosters retention. When the employer is able to create opportunities for advancement and new learning and increase autonomy and recognition for achievement, the practitioner will typically remain on the job. In 1992, the AOTA reported that almost 24% of OTs changed jobs in the previous 2 years (Warnecke & Freda, 1992). This suggests that one out of every four are changing jobs. If the manager can provide an opportunity for job mobility and challenge within the organization, there may not be the need from the practitioners to seek out alternative employment. This can be achieved through various methods. Communicating with the staff about those needs that they wish to have met is a start in retention and sometimes job rotation. Allowing for clinical research opportunities and promoting program development are strategies that enable practitioners to develop their professional interests, thus creating a challenge in the workplace. Self-actualization professionally is what all OT practitioners try to achieve. The manager who is sensitive to this and creates an environment that supports this has more success with retaining staff.

There has been a lot of discussion about maintaining professional competency during the past 5 years. In fact, during the 1996 AOTA conference, the National Board for Certification in Occupational Therapy (NBCOT), formerly the American Occupational Therapy Certification Board (AOTCB), shared the plan for OT practitioners to remain certified in OT. This plan is based on the practitioner demonstrating to the board his or her professional plan for competency. This brings an opportunity for the manager to create opportunities for practitioners to achieve competency by retaining their employment with their current employer. Methods to achieve competency could include independent study, academic coursework, continuing education, teaching activities, research activities, and/or specialty certifications to mention a few (Competency Task Force, 1995). Offering opportunities for demonstrating professional competency can be a retention strategy. Another strategy for retaining practitioners is developing career ladders. A career ladder provides a way for practitioners to gain promotion and increased compensation on the basis of experience, demonstrated confidence, level of participation in continuing education opportunities, and on-the-job training (Gleeson & Wrinkler, 1995). Similar to the recruitment process, a job description clarifying the job duties and essential functions for each position on the ladder is critical. It is also recommended that the relationship to staff in terms of reporting lines and supervision be identified in these job descriptions. Career ladders should be developed with input from the existing staff, administration, and other appropriate personnel. Each step for advancement within each job should have increased responsibility and compensation (Gleeson & Wrinkler, 1995). When developing the ladder, the manager needs to be realistic with the timetable implementation. Developing the criteria and essential functions is a time-consuming step. A study done by Hartford Hospital in Connecticut indicated that clinical ladders provided for differentiation of levels of clinical competence and a motivator for increased responsibility (Kornreich, 1994). As a manager, your ability to enable the staff to be satisfied and move toward self-actualization professionally will help to retain those practitioners in your organization. Because of the retention, quality will continue and a cost-effective tool has been implemented. In this era of cost-effective health care, it is critical for OT managers to understand what fosters staff professional growth and competency that is also cost-effective. This may not only retain the staff, but please the administration. A career ladder can encourage and reward clinical specialization, professional training, and participation in professional competency activity (Daniel, 1989).

During the 21st century, OT managers will need to be flexible and creative as they continue to address the issues of recruitment and retention. It will continue to be important that managers achieve worker loyalty and commitment as the shortage continues for OT practitioners. After all, practitioners are the limited resource managers need to manage effectively.

Questions

1. Job orientation begins:
    a. The first day of work
    b. At the time of the first performance review
    c. During the interview process
    d. At the end of the probation period

2. A job description contains which of the following categories?
    a. Personality characteristics necessary to perform job
    b. Job duties and essential functions
    c. Dress code
    d. Organizational relationships and mission

3. A definition of recruitment is:
    a. Understanding the employee's needs so the job has value to the organization
    b. Selling a job
    c. Maintaining competency
    d. The process of adding new individuals to a population

4. List the seven steps managers go through during recruitment:
   1.
   2.
   3.
   4.
   5.
   6.
   7.

5. Professional networking in the community for the department manager is important for:
   a. Recognition
   b. Recruitment
   c. Retention
   d. Getting ahead

6. Highest shortage for therapy practitioners in the late 1990s:
   a. Is because mergers, acquisitions, and joint ventures will require more
   b. Is due to the need for competency
   c. Will be resolved
   d. Is in acute care hospitals

7. Which of the following is part of the retention process?
   a. Job definition
   b. Performance appraisal
   c. Career ladders
   d. Welcome process

8. The agency responsible for certification of OT practitioners is:
   a. ACOTE
   b. AOTA
   c. AOTF
   d. NBCOT

9. A career ladder is:
   a. A strategy to address retention
   b. Effective in all job settings
   c. Facilitating employees to achieve additional education
   d. Discouraging staff to resign

10. Professional competency can be achieved through:
   a. Specialty certification
   b. Changing jobs
   c. Networking
   d. Productivity

Case Study 1

The OT department in a long-term care facility has six professional and two support staff (4 OTRs, 2 COTAs, 1 OTA, and 1 clerical staff). One of the OTRs is the manager who has 25% responsibility for patient care. The department is offering sub-acute rehab, outpatient services, and home health services. A competitor in the same town has just renovated a wing of its facility providing 1,500 square feet for sub-acute rehab services and state-of-the-art equipment. The competitor has arranged for a contract therapy service to staff the unit. The salaries being offered are about 15% more than you offer. Benefit packages are comparable. Your staff has started talking about this new opportunity. A retention plan is necessary. What would you do first?

Case Study 2

You are the rehabilitation manager at an acute care hospital. The services offered are PT, OT, speech pathology, sports medicine, and industrial rehabilitation. There has been an increase in hand referrals over the past 3 months. There are two other health care providers in the community offering hand rehabilitation. The referring hand surgeons have made it known that if your department had a certified hand therapist (CHT), they would potentially refer all their cases to your rehab department. A new CHT is relocating to the area and has expressed interest in working at your facility as well as the other two providers. What would be your plan to recruit this therapist?

References

Accreditation Council for Occupational Therapy Education. (1998). *Report of ACOTE to the Representative Assembly*. Author.

Competency Task Force—American Occupational Therapy Association. (1995). *The commission on practice. Developing, maintaining, and updating competency in occupational therapy: A guide to self-appraisal.* Bethesda, MD: Author.

Daniel, M. S. (1989). A career ladder for registered occupational therapists and certified occupational therapy assistants. *Administration and Management Special Interest Section Newsletter, 5*, 2.

Dawe, N. J., & Smith, J. (1988). Recruitment and retention: A plan for action. *Administration and Management Special Interest Section Newsletter, 4*, 3.

Gleeson, C., & Wrinkler, L. A. (1995). Managing the 3 Rs in the 1990s: Recruitment, retention, reactivation. *Administration and Management Special Interest Section Newsletter, 11*, 4.

Kornreich, M. (1994, June). Clinical ladders take recruitment and retention to new heights. *Rehabilitation Today*.

Makely, S., & Bamberg, R. (1991, November). *The influence of specific employment factors on the recruitment and retention of allied health professionals.* 24th Annual Conference, American Society of Allied Health Professionals, Minneapolis, MN.

McDonald, R. (1996). Yes, rehab works and you're the reason. *Advance for Occupational Therapists, 12*(18), 44.

Parisi, R. A. (1994). Managing human resources. In K. Jacobs & M. Logigian (Eds.). *Functions of a manager in occupational therapy* (Rev. ed.). Thorofare, NJ: SLACK Incorporated.

Schell, B. (1992). *Personnel management: The occupational therapy manager*. Rockville, MD: American Occupational Therapy Association.

Silvergleit, I. (1992). The three r's of staffing: Recruitment, retention, and reactivation. *Administration and Management Special Interest Section Newsletter, 8*, 3.

Warnecke, P., & Freda, M. (1992). Recruitment and retention: A congruence model. *Administration and Management Special Interest Section Newsletter, 8*(3), 4-6.

Webster's Collegiate Dictionary. (1993). New York: The World Publishing Co.

Answer Key

1. c
2. b
3. d
4. Identification of the position, attracting the applicant, screening, interview, checking references, job offer, and follow-up
5. b
6. c
7. c
8. d
9. a
10. a

CHAPTER 7

Documentation in Health Care

Mary Hayes Whinery, MS, OTR/L, CHT
Wilma Rizal-Bilton, MS, OTR/L
Martha K. Logigian, MS, OTR/L

In the current health care environment, accurate and timely written communication is vital. Although dramatic changes in health care have affected the style, content, and quantity of documentation, the need for it remains the same. The pressure of reimbursement has pushed the way toward paperless documentation, while managed care as well as other payment systems, such as Medicare and Medicaid, have increased the demand for clinical recording as a means of explaining the need for OT services. With these trends in mind, it is clear that managers must have skills in computer documentation, medical record documentation, and reimbursement.

Management Information Systems

OT documentation can be categorized as management or patient related. Management information systems allow managers to process information with better accuracy and in a timely manner. This allows managers to be aware of problems and opportunities much faster, enabling them to devote more time to planning instead of analyzing results. It also permits managers to give timely consideration to more complex relationships and greatly assists in decision implementation. The more closely the system is designed for the specific application of the user, the better the results.

Management information software can be specific purpose (e.g., dedicated to performing a specific task such as managing, accounting, or bookkeeping), or it can be general purpose (e.g., those that are adaptable to a wide variety of tasks such as word processing, spreadsheets, or communications). These have been developed to meet the needs of people whose work involves planning, writing, record keeping, calculating, and communicating.

Word processing programs can have a variety of options such as spelling and grammar checks. For the OT, another useful tool which can be added to the program is a medical dictionary, such as *Stedman's Medical Dictionary,* published by Williams and Wilkins, or Dr. Spell, published by Salient Software Systems.

In an OT department, word processing allows ease of production of needed materials such as an organizational chart, mission statement, scope of care, policies and procedures, meeting records, correspondence, and research papers. Its presence can make many tasks easier and less time consuming for support staff, therapists, and managers.

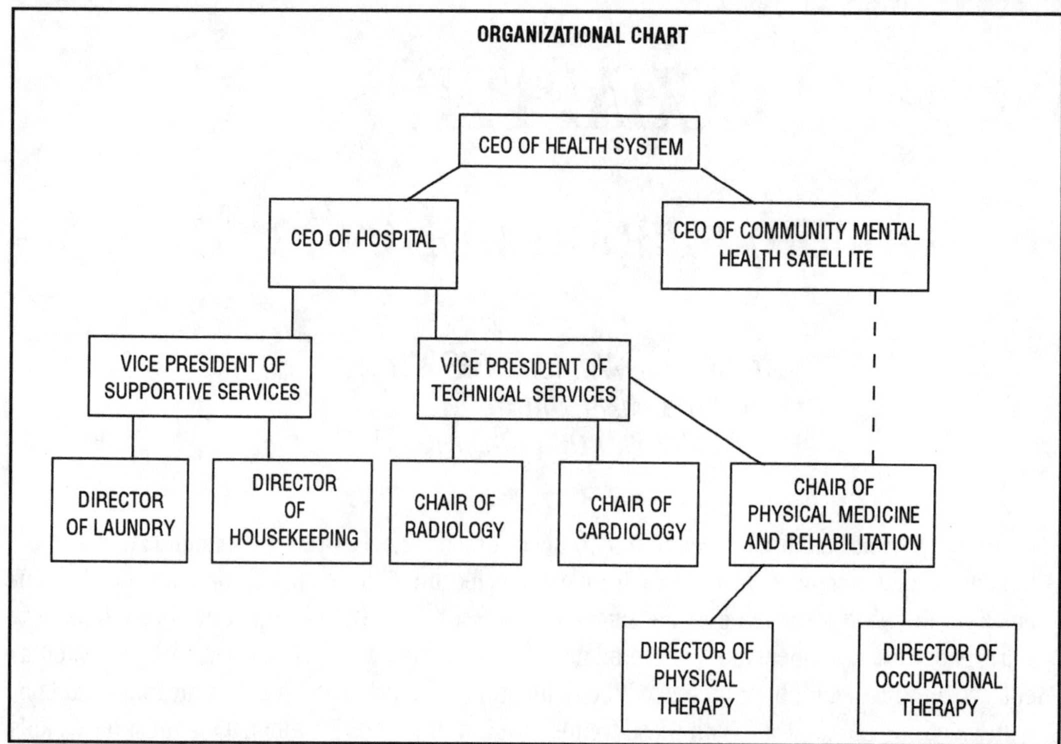

Figure 7-1. A sample organizational chart indicating both direct and indirect lines of authority, responsibility, and communication.

An organizational chart is a graphic representation of the formal structure of an organization or department. It diagrams the lines of authority and communication. The words are positions within the department, while the lines indicate the flow of responsibility. If the lines are solid, they indicate a direct relationship between the positions. Dashed lines indicate an indirect relationship (Figure 7-1).

A department mission statement is consistent with that of the institution. It states the purpose, beliefs, and values of the department and contributes to the definition of the department's scope of care. It is the overall frame of reference or vision of the practice. An example of a mission statement can be seen in Figure 7-2.

The scope of care identifies the target population served, where these services are provided, and defines the clinical activities offered by the department (Figure 7-3).

Policies and procedures (Figure 7-4) ensure consistency in departmental behavior. Policies are guidelines designed to handle recurrent situations, avoid problems, and outline an expected course. Procedures are the sequential steps in the implementation of the policies. They define in operational terms a specific course of action, thus assembling all of the organizational parts. They inform the employee as to what is expected and acceptable. Any consistent information or regulation should be documented as a policy and all staff have the responsibility of knowing each policy. Include known expectations or exclusions, dates the policy is written and regularly reviewed, and organize them into a manual accessible to all staff.

A record of all meetings should be kept in the department. It contains the name of the group, date of the meeting, agenda for the meeting, brief descriptions of all issues discussed, responsible person for follow-up, and specific suggestions/timeline for follow-up.

Mission/Purpose Statement

The OT department of Children's Hospital provides services to those children, from birth to 18 years of age, with neurological and orthopedic conditions. Direct treatment is provided to both in- and outpatients. All services delivered are based on the developmental model.

- Services provided include early intervention and stimulation, physical daily living skills training, sensorimotor learning, developmental activities to promote cognitive and performance skills, therapeutic adaptation, prevention, and family education.
- Consultation is provided to the rehabilitation unit and to the Bay Area school district.
- Children's Hospital has limited its services to the area within a 30-mile radius and will send appropriate referrals to other necessary agencies outside this area.
- The department is committed to the highest level of quality care while recognizing the need for efficiency and cost-effectiveness.
- Treatment is delivered individually or in groups as determined by the children's needs.

The department further defines its mission to include teaching and training other health care professionals, specifically those in the field of OT. It is our belief that the services of Children's Hospital directly benefit the community.

Figure 7-2. The mission or purpose statement of Children's Hospital synthesizes the commitments of the departments.

Scope of Care

Rehabilitation Services provides PT, OT, orthopedic technology, and cardiac rehabilitation for in- and outpatients at the hospital, satellite clinics, and home. The services include exercise, functional and mobility activities, work tolerance, and safety awareness at home. Programs are provided for birth to 16 year olds in the Neonate Intensive Care Unit, Early Intervention Program at Brookside Community Health Center, and Juvenile Arthritis Clinic. Sixteen to 80+ year olds are provided services on inpatient units, recovery rooms, outpatient satellites, and in the home under the community hospice program.

Physician referral is required for all services. Patients are seen within 24 hours of referral receipt. The most frequent patient groups treated are those with orthopedic conditions, arthritis, stroke, neuromuscular disorders, and cardio/pulmonary problems. The level of care provided depends upon the assessment of the individual patient's needs. This includes:

OT:

- Assesses patient's level of function by evaluating self-care skills (e.g., bathing, dressing, feeding, transferring), upper extremity status and positioning needs, and cognitive-perceptual skills and their impact on function and safety.
- Gears treatment to maximize patient's functional independence and safety level.
- Makes recommendations for optimal, safe discharge plan (i.e., need for acute rehab, chronic placement, home services).
- Educates patient's family and other caregivers regarding optimal patient function, safety at home, and splinting.
- Provides a variety of equipment to optimize function and safety in the home environment (e.g., bathroom equipment, adaptive equipment for self-care, splints for upper extremity positioning).

Hand Management:

- Assesses patient's upper extremity function by evaluating range of motion, strength, sensation, and functional use.
- Educates patients/family members/others in wound care, edema control, scar management, sensory retraining, pain management, precautions, and progression of activity level and home exercise program.
- Fabricates splints, scar conformers, and educates patients on wear and care of orthotics.
- Assesses ADL status and makes recommendations for adaptive equipment/techniques to maximize role performance (self-care, child care, home care, work, and leisure).
- Uses modalities, biofeedback, BTE, valpar, and functional activities as adjuncts to therapy.

Figure 7-3. Sample scope of care.

There is a variety of correspondence a manager may utilize, such as a formal letter on letterhead paper from the institution, memorandum, and a variety of reports. A memorandum, or memo, is generally utilized to enhance information flow within a system. This paper trail can be beneficial if used properly as it acts as verification that the information was sent, to whom, and when. The for-

Policy/Procedure
Annual Staff Inservice

Policy:
In order to remain current in the areas of safety and employment health, the OT staff are required to attend the six annual inser vices in the areas of:
1. Body mechanics
2. Verbal instruction
3. Fire and safety
4. Electrical safety
5. Infection control
6. Cardiopulmonary resuscitation

These inservices are conducted by the staff development department.

Procedures:
1. All professionals and OT staff (OTRs and COTAs) are to attend all six required annual inservices. All nonprofessional staff are excused from the CPR inservice.
2. All OT staff are responsible for:
   - Reviewing the monthly education calendar published by the staff development department and posted in the office.
   - Scheduling attendance at each inservice with the clinical supervisor.
   - Verifying attendance at each inservice by signing the staff development attendance sheet.
   - Documenting attendance of each inservice in their individual personnel training profiles, available through the secretary with the date of attendance documented.
3. Noncompliance with this policy will negatively affect annual performance appraisals.

Signed:____________________________ **Date:**________________
Director/Manager

Figure 7-4. A sample policy and procedure for annual staff inservices. This policy consists of title, policy statement, procedures, and result of noncompliance.

mat is concise, explicit, and the content directed to a specific audience. The style usually includes "To" and "From," indicating the name and title of the sender and receiver; "Re," used to identify the nature of the memo; and "Date." The memo is initialed by the sender.

Reports may include monthly activity reports, rationale for productivity statistics, or annual reports highlighting activities from the fiscal year. The last may include goals for the coming year. Another type of report is a proposal or request for a program, personnel, equipment, or space. This should include the advantages or disadvantages of the proposal, a needs assessment, rationale, marketing strategies, and revenue potential.

Memos, correspondence, and reports may be sent on paper or, as is seen more frequently, electronic mail, or e-mail. The benefit of e-mail is that it is transmitted immediately and provides a written record for sender and reader. E-mail lists the names of the sender and receiver and the date and time the communication was written and read.

Spreadsheets are another way the computer can be of use to the manager. They are grids of vertical and horizontal lines into which labels and numbers can be entered to monitor numerical records. A formula is entered that presents the sum of a column of numbers and the computer program calculates and enters the result in the proper position on the grid. In addition, if the numbers change, it will automatically recalculate the new sum. Spreadsheets manipulate numbers the way word processors manipulate words. Each follows the user's directions to perform basic functions (e.g., calculating absolute values, averages, logarithms, and square roots). They take time to set up because the tables and headings must be labeled and formulas defined. Actual figures must be tested in the formulas to ensure that accurate results are produced. Once tested, a template of the matrix can be saved on the disk and recalled for future use. The results can then be printed in tables or graphs. They are ideal to use to monitor productivity of therapists as well as cost per case/treatment. There are many spreadsheet packages available, including Microsoft Excel. This has a variety of features including expense statements, time cards, invoices, and purchase orders.

Database management systems (DBMS) collect, organize, and translate general data into a knowledge bank that can be applied to specific tasks and projects. The system enables the user to structure data into files, sort, compare, and analyze specific data to generate meaningful reports. An example of how DBMS can be used in an OT department is in the ordering of products from catalogues. Files can be made of the name of the catalogue, list of products, page where specific items are found, and price. If a therapist needs to order adapted clothing, the specific information is easily available rather than paging through endless catalogues to find the desired items.

An example of a specific program is Professional File by Software Publishing Corporation. This can be useful in keeping records of patients treated, diagnoses, past medical histories, specific limitations, and treatment plans. This can be especially helpful for research activities. In addition, the AOTA is developing the Centralized Outcome Information Network (COIN), a databank that will link a wide variety of outcomes-related projects such as practice guidelines and service utilization—all useful information for the OT manager. Finally, an essential element for management communication is the modem that can connect the user to a variety of networks allowing communication with peers and access to resources such as medical journals and libraries. Basic to this is electronic mail, or e-mail, enabling instantaneous communication around the world or within an OT department.

For the OT practitioner, there is an information system co-sponsored by AOTA and the American Occupational Therapy Foundation (AOTF) entitled Reliable Source for Occupational Therapy. This is an extensive database that includes OT literature, job bank, and product information, as well as allows access to conferences on-line.

Clinical Documentation

Although documentation reflects the unique character of each facility, there are guidelines of good documentation. Make sure it is organized, clear, concise, complete, accurate, objective, and legible. Rules of English composition, grammar, and spelling must be used (AOTA, 1986). Use plain and understandable language; avoid professional jargon. Only those symbols and abbreviations approved by the facility are to be used in the medical record and writing reports. Include in each entry the date of service and signature of the therapist. Always use good judgment, as information should not be speculative, judgmental, or misleading. Subjective material and personal opinions, if stated at all, should be indicated as such (Skurka & Converse, 1984). The AOTA (1994) has published *Uniform Terminology for Occupational Therapy* that can be useful in identifying common terms for the OT practitioner. The third edition addresses issues of current practice and the parameters of the domain of OT as well as standard definitions. These terms can be helpful in internal documentation, program development, and research, although their application may be limited by specific institutional documentation requirements. This is a particularly important point when utilizing abbreviations. These must reflect the institution's guidelines, not those of the professional organization. The purpose of clinical documentation is to:

- Provide a serial and legal record of the patient's condition and course of therapeutic intervention from admission to discharge

- Serve as an information source for patient care
- Facilitate communication among the health professionals contributing to the patient's care
- Furnish data for use in treatment, education, research, and reimbursement (Ford & Heaton, 1980)

Correct documentation ensures the accountability of the professional and validates the care provided. As a legal document, the medical record is used as justification of treatment on which reimbursement decisions can be made by third party payers. It can be subpoenaed by the court to investigate care or substantiate the degree of progress, ability, disability, or limitation.

Clinical documentation can be found in the primary health record, which is typically centralized, or the secondary record or department working files of worksheets or actual tests. The primary record contains information of the individual's patient care from the health professionals who provided the services. It follows strict procedural guidelines regarding style and content. It is a permanent record of all clinical data affecting the patient in a health care facility (Bruce, 1984). Most OT clinical documentation systems include initial reports or assessments, progress notes, treatment plans, and discharge summaries. Usually this information is handwritten or typed from dictation, although some larger facilities are now using computerized documentation systems.

A referral from a physician is typically required to initiate an evaluation of a patient. This referral is usually required to obtain third party reimbursement. On the referral is stated the patient's name, medical record number, date of birth, date of referral, referral source, diagnosis, pertinent past medical history, precautions, and reason for referral. In some institutions this process is computerized on the doctor's order system. Following receipt of the referral, the therapist assesses the patient and prepares a report (Figure 7-5). Standard information on this report includes the patient's identification information, tests administered, and objective findings. An analysis of specific testing tools may be necessary. Standardized tests should be administered when possible and the results reported in the document. Document a brief summary of the results of all other evaluative procedures with a subsequent OT problem list and recommendations for service addressing each problem. It includes short- and long-term goals written in consultation with the patient and family. Long-term goals are statements of the expected level of outcome at discharge from therapy or the institution. Short-term goals are intermediate steps to achieve the long-term goals. Statements of behavioral objectives or expected outcomes may be required in the assessment note. In the school system, the evaluation report must document educationally related needs provided under the Education for All Handicapped Children Act (P.L.94-142).

A treatment plan is based on the problems and goals with an anticipated time frame for achieving each goal. The development of a treatment plan or plan of care is based on the initial assessment and changed as needed based on reassessments. The plan is updated according to policy and the achievement of goals. It is always signed and dated.

The individual educational plan (IEP) is a treatment plan used in the public school system. It is mandated by P.L.94-142. This federal regulation states that the IEP must be in effect before special education and related services can be provided to a child. An IEP is completed for each child at least annually. It is based on the initial evaluation and ideally developed by the members of the team working with the child. It contains the child's present status, annual goals and related instructional objectives, expected dates of goal achievement, identification of services provided, initiation and duration of the services, and a schedule for determining whether the objectives were attained (AOTA, 1987) (Figure 7-6).

BRIGHAM AND WOMEN'S HOSPITAL
A Teaching Affiliate of Harvard Medical School
75 Francis Street, Boston, Massachusetts 02115

Rehabilitation Services
Occupational Therapy Evaluation

☐ Initial ☐ Discharge

Diagnosis: ______________________________

Orders/Precautions: ______________________________

Social/Environmental: ______________________________

Prior Functional Level: ______________________________

Functional Status/Safety:

Patient/Family Education: ______________________________

Problem List	Short-Term Goals	Long Term Goals
		Treatment Plan

Discharge Plan/Recommendations: ______________________________

Modality/Equipment: ____________ Frequency: ________ Duration: ________

Date: ________ O.T. Signature: ____________ O.T.R./L. Evaluation Time: ________

Date: ________ M.D. Signature: ____________ M.D. Clinician ID# ☐☐☐☐☐☐

FORM # 50668703 Rev 10/93

Figure 7-5. Rehabilitation services OT evaluation. Courtesy of Brigham and Women's Hospital, Boston, MA.

Individualized Educational Plan

Student's Name:	Patricia Green	School:	South Elementary
Birthdate:	2/21/91	Class Placement:	Multi-handicapped
Age:	7 years, 7 months	Teacher:	Mrs. Apple
Date of IEP:	9/11/98		

Student Receives: Speech Therapy __________
Occupational Therapy ____X_____
Physical Therapy ____X_____

Annual Goal (OT):
Improve attentional behaviors.

Short-Term Objective:		Comments:
Patricia will attend to an activity during treatment for 10 minutes, without asking to end or change the activity, once during each daily treatment session.	Begin: 9/15/98 Complete: 10/15/98 Review: / / Achieved: / /	

Annual Goal (OT):
Improve independence in dressing.

Short-Term Objective:		Comments:
Patricia will be able to remove her shoes and socks with minimal assistance at the beginning of the treatment session three out of five times per week.	Begin: 9/15/98 Complete: 11/15/98 Review: / / Achieved: / /	

Annual Goal (PT):
Improve ambulation on stairs.

Short-Term Objective:		Comments:
Patricia will be able to ascend stairs with a minimium of 10 steps, independently with spotting, 80% of the time.	Begin: 9/15/98 Complete: 12/15/98 Review: / / Achieved: / /	

Figure 7-6. An individualized educational plan consists of annual goals, related instructional objectives, expected date of completion, service provided, and initiation of services.

Progress notes (Figure 7-7) reflect attainment of goals and progress, lack of progress, or regression. They generally address the treatment and modalities provided, the patient's response, and amount of time spent with the patient. Changes in treatment plans are stated, as are outcomes as measurable goals and recommendations. Objective data should be used. Attendance is recorded as well as absence including the reason why the patient did not attend. This note can report on activities, dispensing of orthotic devices and equipment, patient and family instruction, and the home exercise program. All notes must be signed and dated by the therapist providing the care. Student notes must be co-signed by a licensed therapist.

When a patient is discharged from OT services, a discharge note is written at the time of the discontinuation of services. It is a summary of the services delivered and recommendations for follow-up. It generally compares the status of the patient at discharge with that of the functional performance on initial assessment. It includes the number of visits, the reason for discontinuation, and the disposition of the patient. Discussion of whether the patient met the short- and long-term goals is included with the date of discharge or last day of treatment indicated. It includes discharge instructions, home program, and recommendations and summarizes any equipment issued. If a follow-up appointment is scheduled, the date and purpose of it should be stated. Also included in the summary is any referral to another agency or community service.

Please sign and date each entry.

Hand Management Note: [ ] PT [ ] OT

Physician Order:

Patient Profile/Precautions:

Procedure/Treatment Plan:
[ ] Fitted with prefabricated splint
[ ] Fabricated custom splint
[ ] Dressing change
[ ] Other:

Modalities:

Equipment Issued:

Patient Education:
[ ] Instructed in wear and care of splint (written and verbal information)
[ ] Instructed in home program of exercise
[ ] Instructed in precautions
[ ] Instructed in wound care
[ ] Other:

Special Issues:

Treatment Goals:

Frequency: **Duration:**

Date: **Therapist Signature:** **Evaluation Time:**

Figure 7-7. Progress note.

Trends in Clinical Documentation

In recent years, every effort has been made to streamline documentation to increase therapist efficiency. Some examples are the use of computerized instruction sheets such as the Patient Instruction Generator. Computerized records are particularly promising as they have the potential to be used with national databases that are useful for outcome studies. An example is Upper Extremity Network (UE Net) developed by the American Society of Hand Therapists in conjunction with Rehabilitation Technology Works and Greenleaf Medical Systems. It was designed to support the goal of a national health care database by the year 2001, to be used in outcome research and in the development of critical pathways. The program uses a personal computer with information being sent to UE Net via a telephone line or local area network. UE Net collects and analyzes the data and provides pooled information to subscribers. Greenleaf Medical Systems has developed the clinical documentation software for UE Net called Outcomes Reporting and Clinical Analysis (ORCA). The system includes a pocket-sized device or Newton that allows the therapist to pen-tap through a progression of clinical screens to document patient data that can be printed. It also includes a patient billing system. Greenleaf has also developed a computerized evaluation system (EVAL) for upper extremity and hand evaluation. The system calculates impairment ratings, evaluates progress, and identifies submaximal effort. A portable version of this called EVAL SOLO SYSTEM is available which includes instruments such as a goniometer, dynamometer, and pinch gauge connected to a compact data control unit which stores patient data.

Occupational Therapy Ethics

Documentation and confidentiality are professional responsibilities supported by the AOTA (1988). Principles of ethics guide professional conduct in the field and direct OTs to conform to local, state, and federal laws and regulations applicable to records and reports. We are obligated to record information as required by the standards of employers and AOTA. If conflict or differences arise among these standards, the OT is responsible for reporting discrepancies to the employer including monitoring for corrective action. AOTA's principles clearly state that objective data govern subjective data in evaluations, recommendations, records, and reports as they are a means of health care accountability. Objective and precise records are a mechanism that relates outcome to therapeutic intervention. The reporting process presents the merits of OT to the client, third party payer, physician, and other health care professionals (AOTA, 1989; Gillette, 1982).

Privacy and confidentiality of patient information is addressed by a number of professional, institutional, state, and federal regulations (Springer, 1971). The OT has the responsibility to utilize all related information solely for the improvement of the client's well-being and safety. Upon request, patients or their representatives are allowed to review their medical record and appeal for changes or corrections. It is generally recommended that the physician or appropriate health care professional be available when the record is reviewed to clarify the information. Therapists should be familiar with patients' rights and remember to use good judgment when writing in the medical record. Release of the patient's record to outside agencies must be approved by the patient or legal guardian. A signed authorization sanctions the release. It is usually available through the medical records department.

Regulations

There are specific rules and regulations for clinical documentation in the medical record. They are often developed by regulating agencies and supported by the medical records department and institutional and professional organizations. Among the requirements are that the patient's name and identification number appear on every page of documentation. Documents must be signed and dated with the health professional's signature of first and last names and designation (i.e., OTR/L, COTA/L, OTS, OTSA). According to the AOTA, all student documentation, as well as that of a COTA, must be co-signed if required by the employer or legislation. The licensing board may require co-signature of notes to indicate some level of supervision. Black ink is used for handwritten documentation to aid duplication and ensure permanence. Typically there is a correction procedure for errors made in the primary record because erasing or covering over the error is not acceptable. It is standard to draw a line through the error, write in the correct statement, and initial the change. When using electronic documentation, the user is given a signature code that is legal identification of the person.

Standards of accrediting and licensing agencies serve as directives for comprehensive documentation. Surveyors are in compliance with these directives when they visit a facility. Each accrediting agency publishes its own standards that are usually updated annually. The standards published by the Joint Commission on the Accreditation of Healthcare Organizations (JCAHO) are those generally used by health care institutions (1996a, 1996b). Medicare guidelines that include documentation requirements are published in the *Federal Register* and are distributed to local intermediaries. As guidelines change frequently, it is essential that therapists be knowledgeable of the current standards from accrediting agencies and those of the local, state, and federal governments.

When participating in clinical research, patients and their families must be informed. An agreement or informed consent that states that the individual understands the risks of the research effort and agrees to participate needs to be signed by the patient. This can also be true for a change in treatment protocol, particularly one in which a standard procedure has been altered or is viewed as experimental.

Storage and retention of the primary health record is strictly controlled. Institutional rules and state statutes stipulate lengths of record retention and handling. If a therapist is responsible for a medical record or part of the health care record, it is necessary to protect it against loss, defacement, and tampering by unauthorized individuals.

The medical records personnel can be particularly helpful with clinical documentation. They are familiar with the current regulations including those of storage and copying. Although traditionally the record is handwritten, the recent trend is toward computer documentation. Nevertheless, before any form or format can become part of the permanent record, it must first be approved by a forms committee usually managed by medical records personnel.

The information in the medical record is the legal communication among health care professionals and is scrutinized by third party payers to determine reimbursement. They rely on the record to justify the need for provision and continuation of care. Members of utilization review committees review the record to determine proper use of services and whether a patient continues to need the specialized care. An organization's quality management personnel monitor patient progress, achievement of goals, and clinical competence from the record (Ottenbacher, 1986).

Documentation System

When developing or upgrading a documentation system, every effort should be made to ensure that all components complement one another. Table 7-1 provides AOTA's considerations for good documentation (AOTA, 1986). In addition, Table 7-1 presents questions that should be asked when designing a system. When all factors are weighed and a system is in place, policies must be written which complement the system. Objectivity, accuracy, and brevity without sacrifice of essential facts remain the hallmarks of effective records. The challenge is to implement a comprehensive and efficient system that meets the needs of the individual department, complies with governmental and third party regulations, and allows the therapist time to provide quality patient care.

Note: This chapter has been helped considerably by the work of two OTs who contributed to earlier editions of this book. We would like to thank Jan Gannon for the chapter on Management Information Systems and Janice Pagonis for the chapter on Documentation. Each made significant contributions to the OT management literature.

Table 7-1
Considerations for a Documentation System

- Is the system consistent within the organization?
- Does the system meet the needs of the organization?
- Does the documentation system comply with the rules of external regulating agencies?
- Is the system approved by medical records, forms committee, or necessary internal group?
- Does the system conform to AOTA's guidelines of documentation?
- Does the system document sufficient information to justify treatment?
- Is the system readily usable by all health care professionals?
- Are the abbreviations used in the system approved by the medical records department?
- Does the system utilize Uniform Terminology?

Questions

1. What is a DBMS and how can it be of value to an OT department?

2. What is a modem and how can it be utilized in an OT department?

3. Health care documentation:
   a. Consists of informational and clinical data
   b. Is patient related
   c. Is located in the primary and secondary records
   d. All of the above
   e. Only a and b

4. Some characteristics of good documentation include:
   a. The language should be clear and understandable
   b. Each entry should be signed and dated
   c. The content should be objective and legible
   d. All of the above

5. Clinical documentation is used by:
   a. Third party payers for reimbursement
   b. Quality management to assess clinical practice and investigate quality care issues
   c. Lawyers to provide substantiating information to support litigation
   d. All of the above

Case Study 1

An OT department was having trouble maintaining sufficient quantities of ADL supplies. Commonly used items, such as long-handled sponges and shoehorns, were frequently out of stock. Large quantities of special supplies were ordered and used by only a few patients. Consequently, many items in the ADL supply closet were obsolete. Running out of supplies caused frustrations for the OTs and patients, yet it was very costly to carry large amounts of excess inventory.

To solve the problem, a formalized inventory system was developed that accounted for weekly/monthly usage of items in the department to provide a sufficient supply to prevent stockouts. To accomplish this task, the managers met to discuss the problem and suggest ideas to resolve it. A successful information system on inventory requires gaining support of the users to acknowledge a need for change and making sure it meets their needs.

The first step in the process was to take a manual count of all ADL supplies—the quantity and variety—in the department to determine which were still relevant and then prepare an inventory supply list. The next step was to evaluate the amount of supplies used each week and the time it takes to order and receive supplies. Next, quantity discounts were explored, and a reorder quantity and reorder point were developed for each inventory item. The reorder point is a trigger point that indicates it is time to place an order when a given quantity of supplies remain in stock.

Once this information is gathered, the inventory system was ready to be computerized. A DBMS program was chosen to allow development of records on each item in stock and specific venders that supplied the products. Files were developed on all products and venders. An example of a product record is:

Product Name:	Elastic Laces
Product Number:	1443
Vender:	Alimed
Unit Discount:	N/A
Unit Cost:	$0.25
Monthly Usage:	150
Order Amount:	200
Reorder Point:	50

This record is part of a product file on all ADL equipment related to personal care. The product files were then grouped together with the vender files to complete the database.

The database was set up as a relational database. This allowed reports to be generated that cross-referenced different files. A report often generated was the list of vender names and addresses with the product name, number, and order amount. This served as a useful reference for the staff member ordering the supplies.

The inventory system saved the department of rehabilitation services $3,000 its first year, reduced the number of stockouts by 20%, and saved time ordering. Most importantly, the quality of patient care was improved.

Case Study 2

You have just been hired as the first OT for a 50-bed rural, acute care hospital and have been asked to develop an assessment tool for patient care. Describe what assessment components need to be included and design the form including room at the upper right-hand corner for the patient addressograph. Take into account the hospital's documentation format, rules and regulations from third party payers and government agencies, and professional guidelines.

Standard information to consider is:

- Initial assessment date
- ICD9 code
- Date of onset
- Physician order
- Precautions
- Patient profile/pertinent medical history
- Prior functional level
- Objective assessment results/physical, functional, environmental, social status
- Problem list/short-term goals/long-term goals/discharge plan
- Treatment plan
- Rehab potential/frequency/duration
- Signature/discipline/time/date

Case Study 3

OTs working in rehabilitation units of hospitals must often design home activity programs for their patients prior to discharge. This is a time-consuming and tedious process. For certain diagnoses, such as total hip replacements, the programs for different patients are often similar. To reduce the time of individual OTs writing home programs, this information is computerized using word processing software.

To start the process, a group of OTs met to discuss the value of such an information system and how it could increase their time to do more active therapy with patients. The first step was to list all the necessary components of a complete home program. Individual OTs were asked to develop sample home programs related to common patient needs, such as range of motion exercises, energy conservation, architectural barriers, and safety. Each program was typed on the word processor to facilitate modifications. They then met as a group to review and discuss each other's proposals. Once the group agreed upon the content of each subject area, the information was finalized on the word processor. A program was designed to allow the individual therapist to pick and choose what information would be given to the patient. All the OT had to do was select the topic relevant to the patient, such as safety in the home, and print out the items, such as bathroom safety. The therapist was also able to personalize the home program by printing the patient's name and address at the top. The program allowed the OT to add specialized instructions as necessary.

The therapists were extremely happy with the success of their efforts. The information system they developed allowed them to produce a professional, personalized home activity program in a short period of time. The system was flexible to meet individual patient needs and was very time- and cost-effective. The information contained in the program could be updated quickly and easily on the word processor.

References

American Occupational Therapy Association. (1986, December). Guidelines for occupational therapy documentation. *Am J Occup Ther, 40*(12), 830-832.

American Occupational Therapy Association. (1987). *Guidelines for occupational therapy in the school system.* Rockville, MD: Author.

American Occupational Therapy Association. (1988). *Principles of occupational therapy ethics.* Rockville, MD: Author.

American Occupational Therapy Association. (1989). *Ensuring payment through documentation: A common sense approach.* Rockville, MD: Author.

American Occupational Therapy Association. (1994). Uniform terminology for occupational therapy (3rd ed.). *Am J Occup Ther, 48*(11), 1048-1059.

Bruce, J. C. (1984). *Privacy and confidentiality of health care information.* Chicago: American Hospital Association.

Ford, R. C., & Heaton, C. P. (1980). *Principles of management: A decision-making approach.* Reston, VA: Reston Publishing Co.

Gillette, N. P. (1982, August). Nationally speaking: A data base for occupational therapy documentation through research. *Am J Occup Ther, 36*(8), 499-501.

Joint Commission on the Accreditation of Healthcare Organizations. (1996a). *Comprehensive accreditation manual for hospitals.* Chicago: Author.

Joint Commission on the Accreditation of Healthcare Organizations. (1996b). *Long-term care standards manual.* Chicago: Author.

Ottenbacher, K. (1986). *Evaluating clinical change: Strategies for occupational and physical therapists.* Baltimore: Williams and Wilkins.

Skurka, M. F., & Converse, M. E. (Eds.). (1984). *Organization of medical records departments in hospitals.* Chicago: American Hospital Association.

Springer, E. W. (1971). *Automated medical records and the law.* Rockville, MD: Aspen System Corp.

Answer Key

1. Database management system
2. Define and discuss uses for a modem
3. d
4. d
5. d

CHAPTER 8

Ethics and Issues in Occupational Therapy

Gail M. Bloom, MA, OTR/L

Why Ethics?

A clear understanding of ethics is essential to obtaining a professional mastery of OT. The foundations of OT are linked with value-based concepts such as quality of life, competency, autonomy, and duty. These basic underpinnings necessitate that the OT acquire a systematic understanding of the profession's underlying values and moral beliefs.

Ethics is the branch of philosophy that concerns itself with morality. Within the domain of ethics are questions of right vs. wrong. It can be emphasized that ethics is primarily concerned with questions. The study of ethics explores questions such as "What is justice? What is meant by equality, independence, free will, and responsibility?" There are rarely absolutes when examining ethical issues.

Classical thinking divides ethics into deontological theories and teleological theories. Both philosophical schools are associated with certain lines of thinking used to decide the correct course of action when confronted with an ethical decision. Deontology (from the Greek "deon" meaning obligatory) is based on the premise that an action is either right or wrong because of the intrinsic nature of that action to be good or bad. Teleology (from the Greek word "telos" meaning end or purpose) examines the consequence of an action to determine its goodness or badness. One is obligated to attempt to attain a balance of good over bad. There is an implication of measurable difference between an action and the alternatives. The presence of qualitative (or quantitative) variables and the ability to separate the whole into its fundamental elements is assumed. It can be useful to subdivide teleological theory into the concepts of ethical egoism and utilitarianism. Ethical egoism promotes that one should do what will produce the greatest good for oneself. In contrast, utilitarianism promotes that one should do what will produce the greatest universal good for a specified group.

"It is wrong to kill" is an ethical principle. Deontological reasoning proposes that it is wrong to kill because the action of taking a life is objectively bad. Deontology is based on the premise that a moral decision to act or to not take action is founded on a universal imperative. Decision making is expressed in terms of what one is obliged to do because of "conscience," "God's will," "natural order," or other ruling obligations. Would teleological reasoning agree with the deontological judgment that it is wrong to kill? The teleological response would depend on the details of the situation and the desired end result. "The ends justify the means" is the most common way of expressing teleological reasoning. Teleological analysis would examine the consequences of the specific incident. For example, the traditional position of the majority in most societies has been that it is right to fight for one's country during war and kill the enemy; therefore, it is a good act to kill...the good outweighs the bad.

Heated debates about medical ethics provide graphic illustrations of ethical decision making. Should euthanasia be allowed? Using deontological reasoning, one can argue that euthanasia is bad because life must be preserved, or one can argue that euthanasia is good because no one should have to suffer. An ethical egoist might propose that euthanasia is a good thing because of personally not wanting to live in pain, or might present euthanasia as bad because of wanting to be kept alive in case of future medical innovations. A utilitarian might argue that euthanasia is bad because generalizations could be made concerning what makes a life worth living (anyone over a certain age might be deemed not worth saving), or a utilitarian might promote euthanasia as good because it eliminates the need to allocate expensive resources such as the cost of professional care for catastrophic illness, thereby stopping a financial drain on families or society.

Moral Conflict and Problem Solving

Ethical theory provides for a mechanism to reach a judgment among choices. Ethical judgment is dependent upon critical and clear thinking. Moral action is dependent upon rational thought. One must think for oneself and not view what seems to be the commonly accepted as necessarily the correct answer. Ethics demands that moral decisions are made not by emotions, but by logical examination of the questions.

The study of ethics promotes critical analysis of questions or issues. Principles or ideal generalized concepts form the foundation from which judgments are made or action is taken. But what if two or more principles conflict with each other? Or what is one to do if one feels morally obligated to take action and if one believes that the action is contrary to the stated ideals of one's group? It is possible to feel motivated to contradictory actions. Moral conflict is the result of mismatched or inconsistent values. Ethical dissonance might be a consequence of a person's internal discord or it might reflect incompatibility between the individual's values and external values.

The basis for ethical decision making should be intellectual inquiry. Ethical problems focus on questions of what one is obligated to do in a given situation. Problem solving should include taking an inventory of the situation-specific factors. Define the problem. What are the details of the events up to this point? Who are all of the involved parties? What are their thoughts and wishes? Are there relevant laws or policies? Judgments made on comparable or similar cases should be examined. Did this type of situation happen before? How was it resolved and what actions were taken? Is there interpretation of law such as a court decision? Are there interpretations of policy such as departmental procedure or association guidelines? Determine all options and the consequences of each choice. List the possible alternatives. What do you realistically expect would happen with each potential course of action? Weigh the competing rights, needs, and interests of the involved parties. What are the positives and negatives associated with each choice? Decide on a course of action or, when appropriate, inaction.

Prioritizing Care: A Moral Health Care Dilemma

Ethical problems focus on questions of what one is obligated to do in a given situation. The health care system has become overburdened by increasing needs and increasing costs. Critical shortages of skilled personnel have alternated with oversaturated professional markets. The OT is faced with increasing demands and decreasing assets resulting in ethical dilemmas related to resource allocation and distribution. Must an OT choose between quality and quantity of care? OTs must give serious thought to allocation in terms of therapist time and, consequently, type and quality of intervention.

The social and financial costs of each case should be included in an inventory of the situation-specific factors in making a determination of whether treatment should be given or withheld. Just as the type of treatment should be based on well-thought-out principles of therapeutic intervention, so should the allocation of treatment be based on well-thought-out ethical principles.

The therapist is confronted with the question of whether one meets the basic needs of many or gives emphasis to the few but most needy. How is the therapist to determine which individuals are "most needy" or which individuals are most "deserving" of treatment? Should treatment allocation be based on prognosis? Or expected quality of life? Or age? Or expense or value to society? Or ability to pay for the treatment? Or productivity quotas? Or probable benefit if treatment is provided? Or probable harm if treatment is denied? All of these options and others have been proposed as acceptable policy. Health care is not a right in our current society. Access to health care (and the quality of health care provided) is determined by public policy.

Payment issues frequently add to the uncertainty. Third party reimbursement guidelines may conflict with therapy treatment goals by in some way limiting therapeutic intervention. Should the OT provide service without reimbursement? Should the therapist seek payment directly from the patient? What if the patient or the patient's family does not have the financial ability to arrange for private payment? Is OT to be provided to only those persons who can afford to purchase it or who have been able to obtain third party coverage?

Traditional medical ethics emphasizes a dual duty to promote good (beneficence) and to avoid harm (maleficence). Serious questions as to the nature of "goodness" arise with increasing frequency. As a society we have not come to a consensus concerning moral goodness. Social change is outpacing social policy because of rapid scientific advancements in technology and medicine complemented by demographic shifts. Enhanced awareness of health risks and better nutrition have contributed to a population living longer. However, there is a corresponding increase in the incidence of chronic or disabling conditions.

Questions such as "Good for whom?" and "Harm who?" gain extra meaning for a society that is rationing health care. Competing interests must be weighed. What are the benefits and costs to the patient, the patient's family, the health care providers, the health care facility, the health insurance agency, society at large? In weighing the options, the OT has an obligation to be aware of the wishes of the patient, relevant laws or regulations, institutional policies, and financial regulations.

Principles Related to Care and Practice

Fundamental questions focus on a patient's right to obtain treatment or to refuse intervention. Legal decisions vary from state to state concerning the withdrawing (stopping treatment once initiated) and withholding (not initiating treatment) of medical interventions. Most of the court cases have focused on life-sustaining measures, and there are strong implications for the practice of OT. (For example, what would you do if a patient with high level quadriplegia requested a long-handled reacher so she could pull the plug on her life-maintaining ventilator?)

One of the basic tenets of medical ethics is informed consent. Informed consent implies that a patient has a capacity for judgment. Historically, the generally accepted standard of informed consent was limited to a description of what was likely to happen to the patient based on the proposed treatment plan. During the 1970s, a new standard of informed consent developed. "Therapeutic privilege" is no longer accepted as a valid reason to withhold information from a patient. Medical professionals acknowledge the patient's right to be involved and to participate in the decision-making process. The OT must include the patient as an active participant in the decision-making process.

Informed consent is based on the principle that the patient must be given sufficient information for a reasonable person to make a decision. The nature and purpose of the proposed treatment must be explained. The foreseeable consequences and the probable risks (as well as less common possibilities) must be presented. Information must be given as to the seriousness of the risks and the degree and likelihood of danger. The patient should be made aware of the rate and probability of successful intervention. If available, treatment alternatives must be presented. The patient must be told about the likely outcomes if the recommended procedure is not followed.

When obtaining informed consent, information must be presented in a manner that will reduce anxiety as much as possible in order to facilitate communication. Jargon and technical language should be defined in order to encourage understanding by the patient. Only the relevant issues (materiality) need to be taken into consideration. "Relevancy" is subjective; therefore, the OT should consider what is meaningful and significant for decision making for this individual in this particular situation.

Competency is a legal standard that defines the ability of an individual to make a free choice. A person might be determined, but not competent, to give informed consent when of minor age or because of a developmental, degenerative, or traumatic incident resulting in disrupted mental status. Court rulings have decided that an incompetent person has the same legal rights as a competent person.

The preferred procedure to protect the rights of an incompetent individual varies on a state-to-state basis. The right to grant or refuse consent for treatment can be reserved by the state court system or can be awarded to a guardian (family member or court-appointed guardian) or a specially appointed team (e.g., a hospital ethics committee). Some states recognize a health care proxy, a family member or friend designated by an individual to make medical treatment decisions if unable to retain the capacity to make decisions. When making a treatment decision for an incompetent person, one must consider if the individual made wishes or beliefs known while still competent. Has the patient made a clear, explicit advance directive? This might have been in the form of a living will or might have been in conversation with a medical professional.

Without advance direction, the decision-making team is expected to do what would be reasonably considered to be in the best interest of the patient. Patient rights must be preserved by following the recommended guidelines itemized in obtaining informed consent to determine what is appropriate on behalf of the individual. Substituted judgment requires looking at an issue from the perspective of the incompetent individual. What would this person want if this person could tell us? The current and potential quality of life of the individual is examined by factoring the anticipated benefits with the expected burdens.

For example, an OT assigned to a patient with advanced dementia and hemiplegia might contemplate the impact of splinting. The alternatives would be considered in terms of thinking "in the shoes" of Mrs. Jones. If I were Mrs. Jones, under what circumstances would I choose to have a splint? What would I do if I realized that a splint could help the functional position of my hand and prevent contractures? What if I knew that the splint would cause pain during the fabrication process? What if I knew that I might accidentally injure myself while routinely wearing the splint? Is the staffing at the facility ample enough to check my splint to prevent skin breakdown? Would the OT fabricating my splint have spent the time with a different patient with a brighter prognosis, and would that knowledge matter to me?

Principles Related to Practice Implementation

Social values organize behavioral norms for group members. Certain kinds of actions are considered praiseworthy or blameworthy. Different groups establish different value systems. Individual group members internalize the social values dependent upon various personal circumstances such as a sense of identification with the group, conflicting group memberships, or the consequences for noncompliance.

An obligation for member compliance to the rules is assumed by each governing body. The standards are a reflection of fundamental organizational principles. Different types of governing bodies have been empowered to varying degrees but each has the right to institute negative consequences or sanctions when rules are violated. Each group assumes jurisdiction over its own constituency.

Custom, ritual, and etiquette are relatively informal value systems that establish the structure of social morality. Some ethical principles have been codified into more formal standards. Each governing body assumes the authority to formulate rules for its own membership. Law, statute, and ordinance are binding rules of conduct enacted by a government. Regulation is instituted by associations or governmental departments, but generally does not have the same power as statute. Policy is considered to be less authoritative than regulation. Guideline is recognized to have less force than policy.

Federal, state, and municipal governments through executive and legislative branches enact laws and ordinances. A municipal government has less direct influence than does a state legislature. A state's Department of Mental Health can promulgate regulations, formulate policies, and issue guidelines. OT licensure and certification boards have regulatory power and can control activities of OTs at the state level. A hospital can develop personnel policies or departmental procedures and will expect employee compliance. Organizations develop rules and standards for their membership constituencies, and they expect membership compliance and sanction corresponding to the appropriate level of influence.

The AOTA, NBCOT, state licensure boards, Medicare, and Medicaid are among the many authorities that regulate the practice of OT. Standards establish minimum expectations of competency. Professional competency can be determined by therapist acquisition of skills and performance on tasks as is recommended by the guidelines provided by the professional agencies. Competent performance is attained with an understanding of the profession's underlying basic moral values. Noncompliance leaves the therapist vulnerable to accusations of malpractice or negligence. Malpractice is action performed not in accordance to the routine and customary standards of the profession. Negligence is inaction that is not according to routine and customary professional standards. Sanctions can vary dependent on the authority of the regulating agency and can include a range from private reprimands to probation to suspension or loss of license to practice as an OT. Some agencies and the courts can levy fines.

In addition to determining basic levels of competency and accountability, state licensure and certification boards can provide other benefits. A primary purpose of OT licensing boards is to protect the public. Consumers are shielded from unqualified practitioners.

As OTs we have a responsibility to be informed about our own rights and obligations as students, employees, supervisors, and employers. We have a professional obligation to develop advocacy skills on behalf of those who utilize our services. It is our duty to be aware of all the laws and regulations relevant to our practices. Additionally, an OT has a duty to be responsive to the duties and responsibilities of the profession expressed in the *Occupational Therapy Code of Ethics* (see Appendix A).

The *Occupational Therapy Code of Ethics*

The *Occupational Therapy Code of Ethics* was written to provide guidelines to all OT practitioners (OTRs, COTAs, students, and OT aides). The *Occupational Therapy Code of Ethics* is an official document of the AOTA and is binding to its membership with sanctions imposed by the Commission on Standards and Ethics.

- OTs are expected to provide services without discrimination.
- OTs must promote the greatest good and avoid doing harm.
- OTs must maintain professional standards, such as obtaining informed consent and honoring the right to refuse services.
- Follow the routine, acceptable operating procedures specified in the AOTA *Standards of Practice*. Maintain a high level of competence.
- Proper billing and business practices should exist. Avoid any activity that is fraudulent or abusive (such as excessive reimbursement requests, charging for services not delivered, inaccurate documentation). Avoid conflict of interest.
- Confidentiality must be respected for those who receive services as well as for colleagues. Report unethical practices to the appropriate authority.

The Americans with Disabilities Act

The ADA is intended to eliminate discrimination against individuals with disabilities. The ADA extends federal civil rights legislation to prohibit discrimination on the basis of race, color, national origin, sex, age, or disability. The intent of the law is to mandate equal access to employment, services, programs, and activities for individuals who would otherwise qualify but were denied participation because of the presence of a disability. The definition to determine if a person is disabled and therefore qualified for legal protective rights is in response to a two-part question:

1. Does the person have a disability, have a history of a disability, or treated as if having a disability?
2. Does the disability limit a major life activity?

Persons who have a history of a disorder and are cured or in remission and persons who give others the impression of having an impairment (even if not diagnosed) have equal protection from discrimination.

The ADA requires reasonable accommodation in the most integrated setting appropriate to the needs of the disabled individual. What constitutes "reasonableness" will not always be clear. Reasonableness requires modification that is not prohibitively expensive or difficult to administer and does not fundamentally alter a program. Reasonable accommodation must be determined on a situation-specific basis. Reasonable accommodations have included the restructure of facilities with ramps, wider public bathroom doors, and modified telephones. Modified work schedules, alternative testing methods, and the provision of qualified interpreters are usually considered to be reasonable accommodations. Facilities are required to become handicapped accessible with new construction or with significant alteration of existing structures.

In considering employment, an applicant has the burden of establishing competence for a position. The ADA requires the employer to determine essential job functions and to consider the consequences of a function not performed. A person will be considered as "qualified" if the essential job functions can be accomplished with or without accommodations. The employer is not required to hire or continue to employ an individual who provides a direct threat to the health and safety of others or to him- or herself unless the risk can be eliminated by providing reasonable accommodation.

Conclusion

OT has a rich value-based tradition deeply rooted in social philosophy. As OTs, we routinely include careful consideration of independence and quality of life in our everyday work.

OT clinicians and managers develop expertise in applied problem solving, proficiency with functional analysis, and understanding interpersonal behavior. These treatment-oriented skills can readily transfer to ethical decision making.

Questions

1. Ethics is the branch of philosophy that is concerned with:
    a. Politics
    b. Morality
    c. Language
    d. All of the above

2. Ethical decision making should be based on:
    a. Logical examination of the issues
    b. Critical and clear thinking
    c. Rational thought rather than emotion
    d. All of the above

3. The *Occupational Therapy Code of Ethics* recommends that OTs should:
    a. Maintain high standards of competence by participating in educational activities
    b. Take all reasonable precautions to avoid harm
    c. Understand and abide by applicable policies; local, state, and federal laws; and institutional rules
    d. All of the above

4. Informed consent is based on the principle that:
    a. Medical professionals should make treatment decisions based on scientific research
    b. Medical professionals should make treatment decisions based on cost analysis and the availability of resources
    c. Medical professionals should make treatment decisions based on the active involvement of the patient in the treatment planning process
    d. None of the above

5. Best interest is founded on the principle that medical professionals should make treatment decisions for incompetent individuals based on:
    a. Cost analysis and the availability of resources
    b. Looking at the situation from the perspective of the incompetent individual
    c. Social consensus
    d. None of the above

6. To solve an ethical problem, an OT should:
   a. Analyze the problem by looking at similar situations
   b. Follow one's best instincts
   c. Determine and follow social consensus
   d. All of the above

7. Not adhering to the customary and routine standards of the profession can leave an OT vulnerable to:
   a. Negligence liability
   b. Malpractice liability
   c. Loss of license to practice as a clinician
   d. All of the above

8. The ADA is a federal civil rights law amended to protect:
   a. Persons with an impairment that limits a major life activity
   b. Persons with a temporary disability that does not limit a major life activity
   c. Only persons with physical disabilities
   d. All of the above

9. An OT who works in a public high school has completed the fitting of a hand splint. Prior to splint fabrication, the OT took time to explain the purpose of the splint, the potential risks, and the probability of success. No guarantees were offered nor were threats made; however, the high school student was told about the likely outcomes if the recommended procedure was not followed. The student agreed to wear the splint. The OT used:
   a. Proper procedure for substituted judgment
   b. Proper procedure for obtaining informed consent
   c. Extraordinary measures beyond what is routinely required procedure
   d. None of the above

10. OTs frequently deal with ethical problems because of:
    a. Increasing demands for OT services and a shortage of qualified OTs
    b. Lack of social consensus concerning medical-ethical questions
    c. Payment policies limiting OT intervention
    d. All of the above

Case Study 1

This was the second admission within a few months for Phyllis, a 72-year-old retired OT.

Medical history included radiation and chemotherapy for neck tumors and esophageal carcinoma. (Dysphagia and weight loss are common symptoms of this type of cancer. Possible side effects of chemotherapy include lethargy and weakness.) Included in the history were recurrent depressive episodes, although last hospitalization for depression occurred years ago. (Symptoms of depression include changes in appetite and sleep patterns, low energy, fatigue, and a constant feeling of sadness.)

On admission, Phyllis presented with low energy, fatigue, and significant weight loss, symptoms that could indicate growth of new tumors, side effects to previous treatments, or major depression. Her primary physician made referrals including comprehensive evaluation (complete medical workup, psychological testing, and OT testing) followed by treatment as indicated by differential diagnosis.

At the next team meeting, the medical team was reluctant to make a firm diagnosis. Refusing to cooperate, Phyllis would not participate in standardized testing. Phyllis had gained a reputation as a difficult patient. The floor nurses described her as uncooperative, demanding, and irritable. She complained about the food and refused to eat. She was too weak to ambulate. Mental status was alert and oriented. Discussion among the team members focused on issues of competency. Was perception of reality impaired by depression thereby altering decision-making ability? Was Phyllis able to make rational judgments based on her actual situation? The team social worker interrupted the conversation by noting that if Phyllis was not transferred back to her nursing home by the next 3 days, then she would be in jeopardy of losing her nursing home bed. Medicaid regulation only allowed a maximum of 10 days payment for reservation of a nursing home bed when the nursing home resident required acute hospitalization.

Following the meeting, the OT decided to visit Phyllis for an OT-to-OT conversation. Phyllis eloquently shared her thoughts about life saying she felt the absence of her colleagues. Having never married and without family, Phyllis made her work her life's focus. Primarily, she missed the feeling of being useful and productive. Additionally, she believed that she experienced social deprivation due to a speech impairment caused by residual damage to her vocal cords as a result of cancer treatment. "Furthermore," she said, "my only remaining pleasure is no longer satisfying. Everything tastes funny ever since they gave me that radiation treatment. There's nothing left for me to enjoy." Phyllis clearly expressed a wish to be able to die in peace. Tearfully, she requested that the conversation be kept confidential.

The OT realized that she was caught in ethical dilemmas. Respond to the following questions as if you were this OT. Justify each answer.

1. Based on the information presented, do you think that Phyllis should be considered competent or incompetent?
2. Does Phyllis have a right to refuse evaluation procedures that might disclose the presence of a life-threatening condition? Does Phyllis have a right to refuse treatment intervention?
3. By not explicitly disagreeing to the tearful request, is there an implied agreement to not share information and is there an obligation to protect a personal confidence? Is there a professional obligation to share the information? Being concerned with Phyllis' welfare and dignity, what should you do?

Case Study 2

Mr. Jones was referred to outpatient OT, PT, and speech therapy in a large suburban medical-surgical hospital. During an OT treatment session, Mr. Jones mentioned that he had received notification of paid costs for PT and speech. OT was not listed on the insurance company statement. Mr. Jones expressed concern, "Will I be responsible for the cost of OT services? I'm on a fixed income and can't afford extra expenses!"

The OT knew that she had submitted charge slips to the billing office for the past 3 weeks. She assumed that a processing error occurred; however, the billing office assured her that the OT slips for Mr. Jones were received and appropriately processed.

At his next session, Mr. Jones brought in another insurance statement. Once again, PT and speech were credited as paid but OT was not recorded. The OT scheduled an appointment with the hospital fiscal manager.

The meeting with the fiscal manager was not going smoothly. He repeated, "We always do the billing in the same way. It's the only way to get reimbursed. If we don't get the insurers to pay, we get stuck with the costs!" The fiscal manager was referring to his long-standing practice of billing third party reimbursement sources including Medicare, Medicaid, and the private insurers such as Blue Cross/Blue Shield. He said, "We always submit outpatient OT services as PT services. Not only that, but we always put recreation costs into the inpatient OT account; otherwise, the insurers deny us payment for recreation. We need every penny we can get because our overall hospital costs are skyrocketing. If the hospital revenue decreased, we would have to look at drastic cost-saving measures—maybe eliminated departments or reduced staff."

The OT described the situation to the director of OT saying, "You know that my loyalty to this hospital is unquestionable. I recognize the importance of fiscal stability and I am aware of the current economic and demographic trends in the changing health care environment. But I'm worried that OT will never be a routinely covered service if third party payers are not made aware of the significant value of OT. How will we receive proper recognition for the services that we are providing? Submitting costs under a more reimbursable label is misleading our patients, hospital administration, and the insurers. What should we do?"

1. What are the ethical issues in this case? What are your alternatives if you were the OT in this case? Considering ethical principles and guidelines, what would you recommend for a course of action, and why?
2. Develop an appropriate policy for the OT department.
3. Design public policy alternatives that could improve the distribution of health care services. Describe the roles that OTs could assume to help change public policy.

Suggested Readings

Americans with Disabilities Act. (1991, July 26). *Federal Register*.

American Occupational Therapy Association. (1994). Occupational therapy code of ethics. *Am J Occup Ther, 48*, 1037-1038.

Frankena, W. K. (1973). *Ethics* (2nd ed.). Englewood Cliffs, NJ: Prentice-Hall, Inc.

Answer Key

1. b
2. d
3. d
4. c
5. b
6. a
7. d
8. a
9. b
10. d

CHAPTER 9

Quality Management

Martha K. Logigian, MS, OTR/L

Quality management (QM) in health care is the systematic effort to determine if care is provided at an acceptable level. It reflects the degree of adherence to standards of good practice and achievement of anticipated outcome. A common approach to assessing quality care has been to establish a program that measures performance to ensure that it conforms to pre-established standards (i.e., decrease variation of a process). In cases where performance fails to conform, providers attempt to improve behavior via change of intervention or improvement in technique or skill.

The concept of QM began in England in the 19th century. In the United States a means of health care assessment was developed using case histories and re-evaluation of patients 1 year after discharge to determine whether care had been satisfactory. In 1918, the American College of Surgeons established a voluntary accreditation process which set minimum standards and guidelines for physicians to review and analyze hospital care on a regular basis (Meisenheimer, 1985; Merry, 1987).

In the 1950s, the Joint Commission on Accreditation of Hospitals (JCAH) established minimum standards of performance for health care institutions. In the 1960s, to ensure that care was reasonable and necessary, legislation was developed that required hospitals to set up utilization review procedures. By the early 1970s, Professionals Standards Review Organizations (PSROs) were developed by Congress to review medical practices and replace utilization review as a means of identifying appropriateness of services seeking reimbursement. PSROs were made up of local practitioners who determined the appropriate level of care for each patient through chart audit, length of stay, and admission criteria. At the same time, private insurance also adopted criteria for appropriateness of care. In the late 1970s, JCAH and PSROs required that medical care evaluation studies be done by hospitals seeking accreditation and reimbursement (Liang & Fortin, 1991).

In the early 1980s, peer review organizations (PROs) were established for physicians, and utilization review committees continued to function in health care facilities, each ensuring appropriateness of services while attempting to contain costs. At this time, JCAH was renamed the Joint Commission on Accreditation of Healthcare Organizations (JCAHO) and in turn has placed greater emphasis on quality assurance. Its focus is multidisciplinary, with standards of care established for all services. All disciplines in the health care organization are mandated to keep track of services in order to determine if they are being performed in an effective manner. In 1992, the term quality assurance was modified to include quality assessment and improvement standards. The revisions place greater emphasis on the role of hospital leaders in assessing and improving patient care, development of appropriate indicators of care, and further clarifies the interdisciplinary nature of the monitoring process (Donabedian, 1988; JCAHO, 1991, 1992).

In addition to the standards established by JCAHO, there are other methods available to determine quality. Program evaluation, criteria mapping, periodic medical review, and profile analysis are among those that have evolved in response to government and accreditation requirements (Williamson, 1988). Industrial models such as benchmarking and outcome measures utilize methods that focus on productivity, profitability, and customer satisfaction. One such model is total quality management (TQM), which transforms an organization's culture enabling everyone to work every day to create an environment of continuous improvement meeting or exceeding customer needs. Among the concepts associated with TQM is cross-functional coordination (i.e., working on key processes using measures that cut across traditional functions such as finance, marketing, and operations). Other concepts are employee empowerment, horizontal structuring, and QI teams trained in problem-solving tools and basic statistical methods. TQM encourages health care institutions to move away from a focus on compliance to standards and refocus on improvement goals in an effort to deliver high quality care. For many reasons, including the magnitude of cultural changes required to become a quality-driven organization, TQM has not been as successfully adopted as it should have been. However, the basic concepts and ideas of the process are sound and form the cornerstone of modern business and management technologies. There has been an increased awareness of the need for continuous improvement. This need has been addressed in business enterprises by turning toward the philosophy of continuous quality improvement (CQI). CQI views problems, and therefore opportunities to improve quality, as having been built into complex production processes and that defects in quality are rarely attributed to employee lack of will, skill, or intention. Even when people were at the root of the defects, the problem is not one of motivation or effort, but poor job design, failure of leadership, or unclear purpose. In CQI, improvement in quality depends on understanding and revising the production processes on the basis of data about the processes themselves in a constant effort to reduce waste, rework, and complexity. The advantage of CQI is that it builds on existing technology as well as uses concepts of TQM such as cross-functional coordination, a scientific approach to problem-solving, customer satisfaction, use of statistical tools and QI teams, and employee empowerment (Berwick, 1989; Higgins, 1993).

In industry there is a relationship between quality and profitability that is quality from the customer's perspective (*The Quest for Customer Satisfaction*, 1996). This concept is particularly critical in the managed care environment. To attract and keep patients within a system, the system must be focused externally (i.e., on the customer) and aligned internally (i.e., systematic performance). To do this, health care institutions are joining fast-moving corporations in shifting their attention to customer satisfaction and using systems thinking or systems improvement (SI) to transform their performance. SI is a management approach that focuses on the interrelationships and interdependencies of the parts of the system. The goals are to improve outcome, customer satisfaction, and quality for staff and reduce cost.

Although TQM and CQI complement SI, the former are more linear while the latter is circular (Krampf, 1995). For example, a CQI team looked into delays in the emergency room. It was believed to be due to a lack of transport to get patients to tests or admitted to a patient care unit. When diagramming the variables, the team discovered there were many related issues, such as specialist unavailability, inadequate space, inaccessibility of the medical record, and inadequate bed control, not to mention customer frustration at long waits to be treated. The entire system in the emergency room needed to be looked at from a fresh perspective, which is where SI plays a vital role.

Managers routinely confront situations whose remedies have implications beyond their work area. To make lasting change in these situations, the utilization of SI has a good chance for success. The first step associated with using SI is to identify the current situation/process needing attention. Next, determine how changing it will benefit your performance, defining the opportunity for improvement in a goal statement. Step 2 involves analyzing the process in more depth including identifying and collecting relevant data and comparing this data to the current system. When developing an intervention strategy (Step 3), it is best to generate multiple strategies and review each strategy against pre-established criteria. Common criteria include cost, time to implement, impact on the system, and cultural resistance. Ultimately a strategy is chosen, as well as implementation alternatives. An implementation work plan is then developed listing specific steps to complete the project. As part of this step the team working on the process then identifies how to measure the results of the new plan. Step 4 includes clarification with the stakeholder as to the best way to present the plan. Prepare the presentation including all the work done in Steps 1 through 3 and present the data collected and the results of the analysis including who participated. Approval for the recommendations in the plan must be part of the process.

Step 5 is the point when the strategy, analysis, and plan are converted into action. Communication with all involved is key so that the implementation goes smoothly and results can be easily monitored. Evaluating the outcome takes place in Step 6. New data are collected and measured against prior data. If the outcome is successful, continue the plan, document the success, and acknowledge all contributors. If the outcome is not successful, identify the reasons why and return to Step 1. The final step is to evaluate the entire process by which you developed the new system. Summarize lessons learned from the use of the SI model, considering how you want to alter the process and what you want to share with the others (Kaplow, 1996).

Most health care organizations use the QM systems delineated by JCAHO which encompasses CQI methodology. CQI concepts enhance the current 10-step quality monitoring and evaluation process used by JCAHO (Figure 9-1) by establishing a framework for a systematic, ongoing, problem-focused, performance measurement system (Logigian, 1993). This is a shift away from individual departmental and service focused QM toward a generic system that reflects the entire institution.

Critical to this framework is a clearly identified institutional plan for quality patient care. This plan mandates the same level of care throughout the institution. In turn it reflects the needs of both internal and external customers of the institution. Much of the information that is currently required by customers is data intensive, resulting in a reporting system that is costly, inefficient, and typically lacks focus for identifying actions for improving performance. A shared structure reflects reporting of quality measurements in an efficient manner.

In a facility using CQI everyone from top management to service workers and focus groups take responsibility (Step 1), although it is common practice for the manager of a given area such as OT to have overall responsibility in that service. Assisting in the CQI process provides a greater understanding of the findings. Staff who assume ownership are better able to integrate solutions into day-to-day practice.

The second step is to delineate the scope of care. All primary functions of the OT service should be identified (i.e., types of patients served; care delivered such as diagnostic, therapeutic, and preventive services; age groups of patients; basic clinical activities of practitioners; and a definition of who provides care/services). For example, the hand management service provides care for adult patients with hand injuries in an ambulatory clinic, Monday through Friday, 8:00 a.m. to 5:00 p.m. The staff is comprised of hand surgeons and OTs.

Step 3 identifies the important aspects of care provided (i.e., care which occurs frequently, is high risk, or problem prone). Among the primary objectives of an institution-wide effort is to define a set of core quality outcome measures for the processes of care within the institution's committees and departments. For example, in an acute care OT department, services that have high volume would be services that affect large numbers of patients (e.g., safety assessment and functional training for elderly patients living alone). An example of a high-risk service is splinting (i.e., the patient is at risk for developing skin irritation or pressure areas). Problem-prone care are those aspects of care which can already be identified as frequently problematic (e.g., lack of compliance with the treatment regime such as missing scheduled treatment sessions).

In Step 4, indicators of quality are developed. Indicators are defined as measurable dimensions of a specific aspect of care identified in Step 3. Indicators emphasize the appropriateness of care and outcome. This may include the adequacy, timeliness, and effectiveness of an aspect of care. Examples of indicators are seen in Table 9-1.

In Step 5, criteria or thresholds are set to determine how each indicator will be measured (i.e., what percentage or number of instances are acceptable to indicate quality care). The threshold set to measure the safety assessment indicator in Table 9-1 is 85%. In other words, the expectation is that a safety evaluation is performed on 85% of all the elderly patients referred to OT who will return home alone.

The next step is to collect and organize data for each indicator. Using Example 1 cited in Table 9-1, the patient medical record would be utilized for data collection. The medical record is a useful tool when monitoring indicators of care such as accurate and thorough documentation of functional training. Typically, there are four steps to the process:

1. Establish the standards of care to be provided.
2. Charts are reviewed to determine if practice meets the standards.
3. Charts that do not meet the standards are analyzed to identify issues, remedial action is taken, and feedback given.
4. Follow-up is done if indicated by the findings.

Once data are organized, indicators that reach or exceed the pre-established threshold are evaluated to determine the area of concern (Step 7). A new, more specific monitor may be developed to assess the problem. For example, the acceptable threshold for the indicator, hand management referral (see Table 9-1, Example 2), is 95%. The incidence of no referral for a given quarter is found to be 10%. Two new indicators are developed to determine the cause. One indicator monitors the lack of referral due to change in clinic medical staff in the summer (new fellows and residents); the second indicator monitors those due to lack of available appointments in hand management. At the end of the next quarter, data reveal that there is a long waiting time for follow-up appointments which results in patients not appearing for the appointment.

When the problem has been evaluated, action must be taken to resolve the problem (Step 8). To continue the example of hand management referral, a task force is established to examine the wait time for follow-up appointments and make recommendations to resolve the situation. Additional appointment times are established as recommended. Other action strategies may change behavior or identify the need for additional knowledge.

Table 9-1
Quality Management Monitoring

Important Aspects	Indicators	Threshold	Methodology
1. Safety assessment, functional training, and documentation	Appropriate, timely, and accurate safety assessment, functional training and documentation as evidenced by: 1. Safety assessment 2. Documentation of functional training and discharge planning	85%	1. Quarterly random chart review of 20 records by OT 2. Reports to OT director, QM committee, hospital administration
2. Hand management referral	Appropriate, timely, and accurate referral to hand management as evidenced by: 1. Physician order, signed and dated on all post surgical hand patients 2. Postop splinting on day of referral 3. Follow-up treatment within 1 week of receipt of referral	95%	1. Quarterly chart reviewed by hand management service 2. Reports as stated above

In Step 9, the effectiveness of the action taken is assessed and the findings are documented. When the indicator hand management referral is monitored for the next quarter, and the threshold of 95% is not exceeded, it is determined that the task force has resolved the problem.

The last step, communication of relevant information, is the responsibility of the OT director. Typically, QM reports are sent regularly to the administrator of QM and appropriate committees. Table 9-2 provides a suggested outline for how the report may be written. The QM department may choose to make recommendations to other departments or key people as indicated by the findings presented. Most importantly, findings and follow-up must be shared with staff members. This can be done through staff meetings, individual meetings with staff involved with the project, and written communication summarizing the findings with recommendations for future QM activities. Figure 9-1 presents a schematic diagram of this 10-step monitoring and evaluation process.

Measures of quality must emphasize processes, not individuals. Process measures that focus on compliance with procedures do not necessarily reflect all aspects of quality patient care (Kleefield, Churchill, & Laffel, 1991; Laffel & Blumenthal, 1989). In fact, the current changes in the JCAHO standards emphasize the need to assess QI in patient activities, such as the process by which patients are discharged. This is a departure from a discipline-specific, problem-oriented approach to one that emphasizes the integration of efforts to improve patient outcome. In this regard, effort must be directed at institutional leadership to take the lead in QI process.

Time and resources must be substantively invested in the quality care effort which demonstrates respect for health care workers. An open dialogue between customers (patients) and suppliers (health care providers) must be maintained. The focus of QI is on the customer. The institution must be organized for quality, using new managerial techniques that focus on the role of regulators to one of partners with caregivers in developing measurement tools used to evaluate QI. Health care professionals, including physicians, must take an active role in specifying preferred methods of care. Developing clear, scientifically grounded, continuously reviewed statements of

Table 9-2
Guidelines for Documentation of Quality Management Activities

Indicator:	Identify the aspect of care and clinical indicator being discussed.
Evaluation:	Identify the threshold, standard of acceptable care, and actual performance. Outline what has been gleaned from the investigation of the issue.
Recommendations:	Describe what is being recommended to address the areas of concern identified through the review. If no recommendations are made, this should be stated.
Actions:	Describe the steps to be taken to ensure that recommendations are followed. Assign responsibility to a specific person or task force. If no action is necessary, this should be stated.
Follow-Up:	Document plans to ensure that recommendations are followed and that these actions effectively address the issues identified. State the time frame for follow-up.

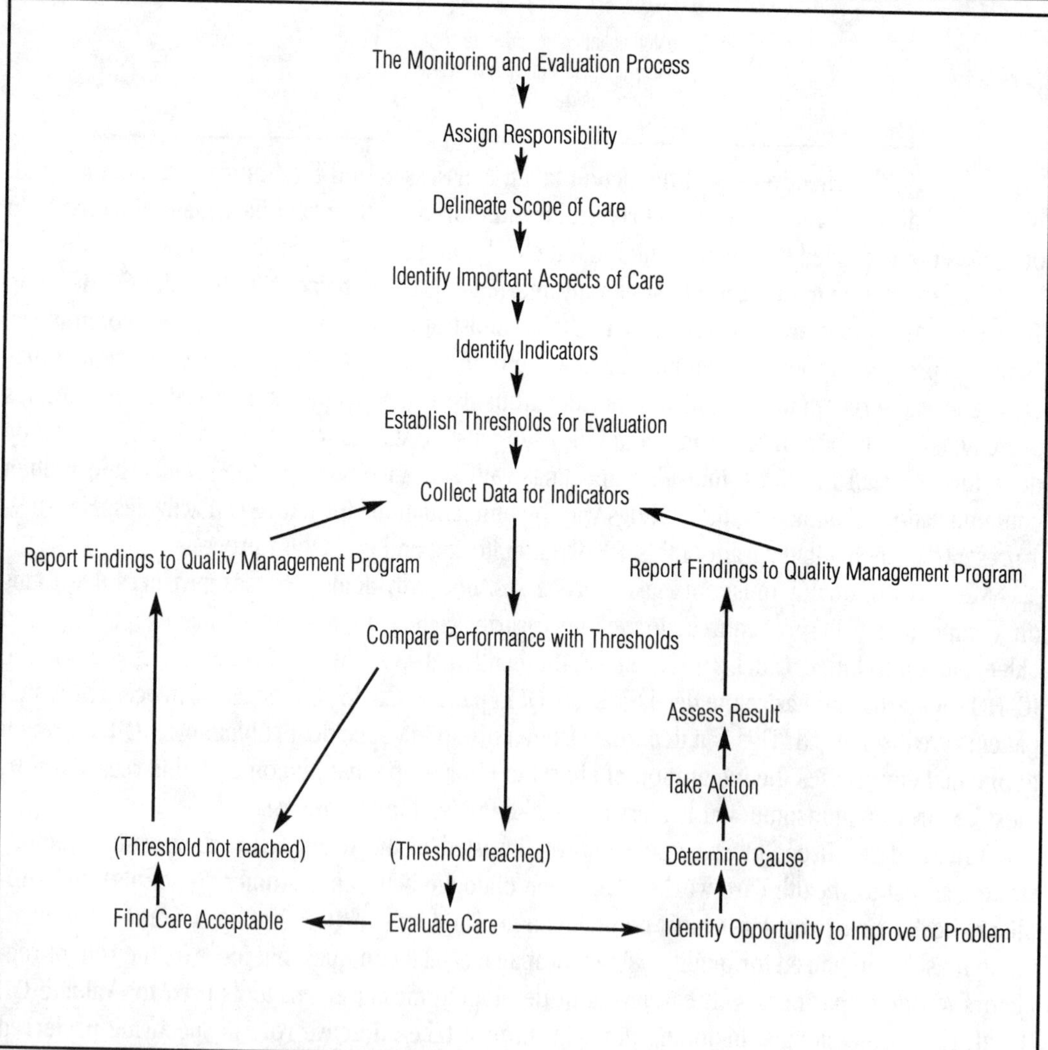

Figure 9-1. QI monitoring and evaluation process.

process (how one intends to behave) are critical to QI. The key is to implement CQI hospital-wide, including physician office practices (Berwick, 1989). The success of QM is based on how well quality care activities are conducted. Simply complying with regulations is not enough. Quality care findings must be meaningful to each practitioner. Current quality care practice is by no means the final step in the continually changing process to adequately define and measure quality care. Awareness of the legal and ethical issues that impact current health care practice is critical. Future QM must ensure that quality results are a balance of these concerns as well as that of fiscal accountability.

Questions

1. When did the concept of QM become organized?
    a. 1950
    b. 19th century
    c. 18th century
    d. 1960

2. PROs were established to:
    a. Ensure appropriate services
    b. Control cost
    c. Both a and b
    d. None of the above

3. Using CQI, the first step is:
    a. Delineate the scope of care
    b. Assign responsibility
    c. Establish thresholds

4. The third step in CQI is:
    a. Establish thresholds
    b. Establish indicators
    c. Establish important aspects of care

5. Once data are organized, indicators that reach pre-established thresholds are:
    a. Evaluated to determine the area of concern
    b. Reviewed by the responsible person
    c. Discussed by the entire organization

6. Measures of quality must emphasize:
    a. Individuals
    b. Processes
    c. Both a and b
    d. None of the above

7. Once data have been collected for indicators:
    a. Findings are reported to the chief of staff
    b. Findings are reported to the clients
    c. Findings are reported to the QM program

8. Indicators may include:
   a. Problems within the department
   b. The concerns of the manager
   c. Specific aspects of care

9. Follow-up should occur:
   a. Whenever the manager has time
   b. Whenever the CEO asks for it
   c. Within a specific time frame

10. A threshold is set between:
   a. 0% to 100%
   b. 80% to 90%
   c. 90% to 100%

Case Study 1

As the new director of OT, you have been asked to develop an action plan to implement a QM program in the department. Using the following questions, prepare your report.

- What is the scope of care for the department, including for whom the care is provided?
- What are the most important services the department provides (key functions or aspects of care)?
- What measures do you use to assess the performance of the important aspects of care?
- What threshold will be set for each measure (indicator)?
- Is this indicator so important that a threshold be set for 100% or 0%?
- What data source will you use for each indicator?
- Who collects the data?
- How do you plan to distribute the results of the data collection?
- What routine follow-up will be planned based upon the findings?

Case Study 2

Mary Brown is the manager of the hand therapy service in an outpatient clinic. There are five hand therapists treating approximately 150 clients per week. Of these clients, 50% need a wrist resting splint. The type of resting splint the service had always used was a prefabricated model that takes 15 minutes to adjust. To help expedite the time it takes to adjust the splints, Mary decided to use another model that the manufacturer said needs no adjusting and costs less per splint. Four weeks after implementing the change in the splint utilized by the service, Mary began to receive complaints about the new splint. Initially, the complaints were that the splint required modification to fit appropriately, taking the therapist at least 10 minutes for each adjustment. The clients began to say that the splint was uncomfortable when worn for more than a few hours. Finally, a frail elderly woman came into the clinic with a hand laceration from the splint she received 2 days earlier. What should Mary do to address this issue of quality control?

References

Berwick, D. M. (1989). Sounding board: Continuous improvement as an ideal in health care. *N Engl J Med, 320*(1), 53-56.

Donabedian, A. (1988). The quality of care: How can it be assessed? *JAMA, 260*, 1743-1748.

Higgins, C. (1993). Quality. *AOTA Administration Management Newsletter, 9*, 1.

Joint Commission on the Accreditation of Healthcare Organizations. (1991). *Quality improvement for hospital clinical and support services*. Chicago: Author.

Joint Commission on the Accreditation of Healthcare Organizations. (1992). *Accreditation manual for hospitals.* Chicago: Author.

Kaplow, H. (Ed.). (1996). *How to get things done. Analytic/systems thinking learning center.* Boston: Brigham and Women's Hospital.

Kleefield S., Churchill W. W., & Laffel G. (1991). Quality improvement in hospital pharmacy department. *QRB, 17* (5), 138-143.

Krampf, L. (1995). Management strategies. *OR Manager.*

Laffel, G., & Blumenthal, D. (1989). The case of using industrial quality management science in health care organizations. *JAMA, 262*(20), 2869-2873.

Liang, M. H., & Fortin, P. (1991). Quality assurance and audit: Lessons from North America. *Annals of Rheumatology Diseases, 50*, 522-525.

Logigian, M. K. (1993). The development of a quality assurance program. *Rheumatology Review, 2*, 87-91.

Meisenheimer, C. G. (1985). *Quality assurance: A complete guide to effective programs*. Rockville, MD: Aspen Systems.

Merry, M. D. (1987). What is quality care? A model for measuring health care excellence. *QRB, 9*, 298-301.

The quest for customer satisfaction. (1996). In W. Leebov & G. Scott, *Service Quality Improvement: The Customer Satisfaction Strategy for Healthcare*. New York: Harper and Row.

Williamson, J. W. (1988). Future policy directions for quality assurance: Lessons from the health accounting experiences. *Inquiry, 25*, 67-77.

Answer Key

1. b
2. c
3. b
4. b
5. a
6. b
7. c
8. c
9. c
10. a

CHAPTER 10

Developing a New Occupational Therapy Program

Mary Jane Youngstrom, MS, OTR/L

Introduction

When faced with the task of conceptualizing, developing, and proposing a new program for an OT department, the manager's initial response may be one of confusion and indecision. Where do you start? How do you think of feasible ideas for programs? What information do you need to support the establishment of a new program? How do you convince administration of the importance of the program and gain support for its implementation?

These are all important questions, and ones that need to be addressed within the program development process. Taken as a whole they may appear overwhelming, but approached in a step-by-step manner, each question becomes an important stage in the overall process of program development.

The What, Why, and Who of Program Development

What is a program and what is program development? A program is a specifically designed service that is aimed toward a specific goal and is designed to achieve clearly defined outcomes or results. An OT department may have numerous programs within the department itself such as a stroke program, a developmental assessment program, or a community re-entry program. The department may be the only provider of service in a program or it may be a participant in a program that includes service providers from several disciplines. Program development is a step-by-step process that focuses on the planning and development of an idea that will lead to a new service in an OT department. It may be as limited as developing a new service in an already established department, such as starting a group feeding training program in a hospital's rehab unit. Or, it may be as comprehensive as designing a program of OT services in a newly opening psychiatric hospital or outlining OT service to be provided for a managed care plan.

Why are programs needed? Programs are needed to clearly focus effort and activity and to directly meet the needs of identified groups. When activities are organized into programs they often become more visible to other groups and help to increase understanding and utilization of OT services. For example, in one OT department, arthritis patients were referred for treatment on an inpatient basis but were rarely referred as outpatients. The department organized an outpatient arthritis program, clearly outlining treatment services and what outcomes patients could expect. When physicians understood this program outpatient referrals increased.

OTs in management and staff positions are frequently faced with the need to develop new programs. The impetus for a new program may come from others, such as when the hospital board of directors decides to open an outpatient arthritis center and the OT manager is asked to develop the OT program for the center. Often the need for a new program will be recognized by an individual therapist, based on his or her day-to-day experiences with patients. An example would be when a therapist recognizes that his or her patients are not improving in their feeding skills as anticipated and decides to develop a special group mealtime program.

The rapidly changing health care environment may also encourage the development of new programs. Developing technology and advances in treatment techniques may prompt new programs. Within the past 20 years, significant advances in hand surgery techniques have fostered the development of specialized post-surgery hand therapy programs. Changes in patient populations admitted to an institution and identification of new diseases such as AIDS have prompted therapists to devise programs to meet the needs of these populations.

Lastly, sometimes new programs are developed to bring together services for clients in a new or more refined way that is more readily understood and accessed by the community. For example, an OT department may have provided preschool screenings on a sporadic basis, but after developing a specific preschool screening program was able to target more schools and provide an increased number of screenings as well as follow-up consultation.

Who does the planning? The planning may be carried out by one person or a group of people. It is often helpful to involve several people or even a committee in the planning process in order to solicit a broad range of ideas and gain differing perspectives. In an OT department the manager or director often carries the official responsibility for program development. However, the responsibility for program development belongs to each therapist who identifies a need for change or sees an opportunity for improving patient care. Official responsibility for the development of a specific program may be delegated to a supervisor, senior therapist, or assigned to a committee. Including others in the development process is advisable in order to increase awareness of OT's role and acceptance of the proposed changes.

Overview of Steps

What does the OT do when faced with the prospect or need for starting a new program? Although initially it may appear to be an insurmountable task, the development of a program is a step-by-step process not unlike the treatment planning process—and therefore one familiar to OTs.

When does program planning and development occur? It can occur at any time—more specifically when a need for a program change is noted. In some organizations planning cycles are formalized so that the opportunity for submission of new program ideas occurs at a routine time. This time is most often connected with the budget cycle. In other organizations a program proposal may be submitted at any time.

The program development process begins with an idea and ends with the implementation of the proposed program. In between these two points the planners engage in an objective and thorough analysis of the actual need for and justification of the program. The specifics of the program are outlined and described, and the costs and benefits of the official program are identified. The steps of the process can be conceptualized as pictured in Figure 10-1. A description of each step follows.

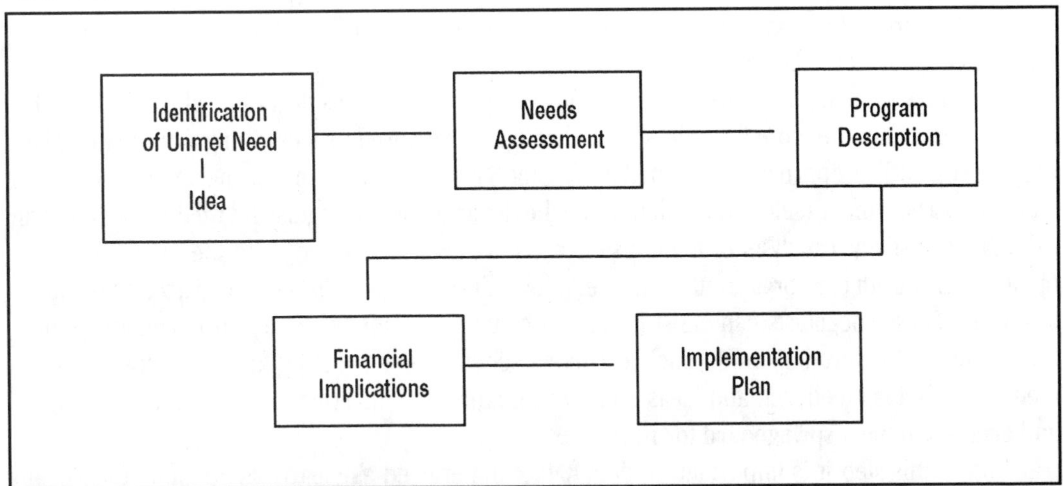

Figure 10-1. Steps in the program development process.

Step 1—The Idea

Ideas for new programs generally spring from the recognition of an unmet need. The therapist who scans his or her environment and listens to and observes what is happening around him or her will discover many sources for ideas.

Patients and their families often know better than anyone else what their unmet needs are and are an excellent source of ideas. By watching patient responses and listening carefully to their concerns, the therapist can often identify the underlying needs being expressed. The therapist who repeatedly listens to the spouses of his or her stroke outpatients express worry and concern about the ability of the husband or wife returning to driving would be using this approach. After listening to their concerns the therapist might identify a need for improved information about driving ability to be made available to patient and family. The therapist might propose that a specialized driving assessment program be developed to address this need.

Feedback from other health care providers can also prompt new ideas for programs. The nurses who repeatedly report to the OT department that patients are not following through with independent feeding skills after the initial OT training may prompt the department to consider a noon time group feeding program.

The community and its members are another source of ideas for new programs. Reading the newspaper and talking to individuals outside of the health care environment can broaden one's perspective and stimulate creative thinking. Involvement in school, church, and community groups can open doors to ideas as well as collaboration. For example, repeated informal contacts with preschool teachers in the community may reveal a need for formal developmental testing—a service an OT could provide.

Critically observing what is currently being done in a department or within one's practice can also provide clues as to unmet needs and ideas for new programs. Analyzing information routinely collected in your department such as attendance/discharge records and CQI reports can lead to ideas for new programs. For example, a QI monitor which looks at amount of improvement in basic self care skills and which documents a low rate of improvement in dressing skills may prompt a department to start a special bedside dressing program. Likewise, analysis of outpatient attendance records which shows poor and irregular attendance by chronic obstructive pulmonary disease patients may prompt a department to establish a more structured 8-week program using a group format to improve attendance and participation.

Ideas may spontaneously arise from various everyday contacts as described above or ideas for a new program may be more formally sought through a structured process using a marketing planning approach. This approach is outlined in Chapter 3 of this book on marketing and includes both an internal assessment (self-audit to determine the department's strengths and weaknesses) and an external assessment (analysis of the consumer, other service providers, and the overall environment). Many health care organizations now employ marketing specialists who can act as a resource to the OT. These specialists can assist in market analysis and identification of potential new programs. Other structured methods, such as surveys sent to patients, family, and/or health care team members soliciting feedback and ideas on new programs, and interviews with key referral sources and clients, can be a springboard for new ideas.

During this step it is important to identify the unmet need as clearly as possible. Clearly but briefly describe the target population, the problem or unmet need, and the proposed program.

As the idea begins to form the program planners also need to ask themselves, "What is the program's overall goal? What is the general thrust of the program?" Defining a goal, even at this early stage, will help to focus the purpose and direction of the program and will guide later steps in the process. For example, an OT department may decide to develop a work hardening program. Is the goal of the program to offer expanded services to current outpatients who are not returning to work quickly, or is the goal to offer a service not readily accessible in the community to a broader population? Depending on the goal chosen, the target population and program scope and design may be very different. The goal selected at this stage is only tentative and may be modified and changed as more information is gathered.

The proposed program and its goal must be compatible with the organization's overall direction and mission. A program that is not compatible with the organization's purpose will never be fully accepted or successfully supported in the sponsoring organization. As an example, an OT department in an acute care hospital decides that a stress management/wellness outpatient program is needed in their community. The mission of the hospital has been defined as providing state-of-the-art medical care to acutely and chronically ill community members. The OT department is able to gather community support and even demonstrate through a survey a strong interest among community members. However, a comparison of the hospital's mission statement with the program's goal shows that the two are not compatible. The hospital's mission is to serve the acutely and chronically ill. The OT department's proposed program is directed toward serving the well community.

Clear definition of the target population, the problem, the broad program solution, and its initial goal prepare the way for Step 2.

Step 2—The Needs Assessment

The purpose of this step is to factually substantiate the need or problem you have identified in Step 1. The following three questions need to be answered:

1. What is the event of the given problem? How many individuals does it affect? How frequently does it occur? Is it expected to increase?
2. How and to what degree is this problem being addressed currently within the department or by others?
3. What are the factors that contribute to or sustain the problem?

The difference between the answers to questions 1 and 2 is the unmet need and will define the extent and size of the problem. The answer to question 3 will support whether your program idea directly addresses one or more of the factors contributing to the problem.

The planners begin by collecting data that specify the size and scope of the problem. Sources of data might include departmental records, medical charts, and/or results of surveys and QA studies. Interviews with individuals in the targeted population to be served or with primary referral sources who would use the new program can contribute to defining the extent and nature of the problem. Demographic information, such as age, rate of occurrence of health problems, and health status indicators, is often available from health care regulatory agencies. Such data can be used to document the extent of the problem or of the targeted population. In the proposed driving assessment program example referred to earlier, the planners would want to identify how many patients treated in the last year would have been potential candidates. A survey of physicians requesting estimates of the number of patients they see per year who might be referred to the programs could also be taken. Both numbers would give planners an idea of exactly how many people might use the proposed program.

The existence of the problem needs to be supported by objective evidence such as statistics and figures that substantiate the level and frequency of occurrence. However, planners should not neglect to use statements of support from prospective clients or program users as well as other organizations or community groups who would agree with the need for the program.

It is important that the needs assessment take place as a separate step in the planning process. Having to substantiate a fledgling program idea with hard data will either convince or dissuade the planners of the need for the program. Without this step, which often acts as a "reality check," planners may proceed with more detailed program development and finally program implementation only to find that the program fails because the need was not as large as was anticipated. The process of gathering real facts about the extent of the problem can also lead the planners to modification of the original program idea which more directly addresses the actual need and will end up being more successful.

When the needs assessment is completed, all the information and data should be analyzed. An accurate picture of the existing situation should emerge. The planners at this point determine if the facts support the need and if the need is large enough to justify spending additional time and resources on further program development planning. Assuming that the answer is yes, the planners proceed to Step 3.

Step 3—The Program Description

During this step of program development the program is outlined and described. The planners must take their idea and describe how the program will work and who will be involved. The overall scope of the program must be defined. The following six topics should be addressed:

1. **Goals and objectives.** The goal initially selected in Step 1 should be re-evaluated in light of all the data collected in the needs assessment step. Does the data collected in the needs assessment support this goal? Or does the general goal and direction of the program need to be modified?

   Once the goal is redefined, program objectives must be formulated. A goal statement for the program, which describes the general thrust of the program, has already been formulated. Now objectives, which are more specific and detail the results and outcomes to be achieved, need to be identified. Objectives a) should be relevant and related to the problem/need identified, b) should be stated in terms of results or outcomes of the program, c) should be measurable, and d) should be achievable. Some examples of goals and objectives for several different programs are described in Table 10-1.

2. **Target population.** The specific population who will be served by the program should be described. Who exactly is the program to serve? Who should not be served? Factors to consider might include age, diagnosis, ability level, and location.
3. **Setting.** Where will the program take place? Will it take place in the hospital or the community? Is the space already allocated or will additional space need to be found? Briefly describe the basic physical requirements of the space needed (e.g., a large open room, three small office spaces, etc.).
4. **Outline of program activities.** A detailed description of the activities and/or methods that will be used to achieve the objectives should be developed. What services will the OT department provide? Does the program include consultation, evaluation, and/or treatment? Will educational activities with family and/or other team members be included in the program? The development of a flow chart detailing how the services will be organized and outlining how a patient will "flow" through the program can be a helpful tool in this process.
5. **Volume.** Based upon the extent of need ascertained during the needs assessment, the demand for service to be provided by the program must now be projected. Volume or service demand frequently varies from month to month. Projections may be made on a monthly basis and plotted out for the first year of program operation. Typically volume for a new program will start out low and gradually increase as the program becomes established and recognized. In predicting volume it is important to be positive yet realistic. Volume projections can end up influencing the program's financial viability and acceptance.
6. **Resource utilization.** After the planners have outlined the activities and estimated the volume of work expected they are in a position to outline the resources the program will require. Resources include space, equipment, supplies, and staff.
   - Space—The proposed program may be housed in existing space, renovated space, or new space. The approximate square footage required and the general type of space needed should be delineated.
   - Equipment—Equipment is categorized into two types: capital equipment and non-capital or minor equipment. Capital equipment is generally considered to be any large item costing $500 or more that will last 2 years or more. Items such as desks, file cabinets, treatment tables, and some test kits are capital items. Smaller equipment items such as hand tools and adaptive equipment are non-capital items. Equipment needs will vary depending on the type of program and the volume anticipated.
   - Supplies—Supplies include all expendable items such as office supplies, test forms, splinting materials, and media supplies. Supply needs will also vary depending on the type of program and volume anticipated.
   - Staff—Two decisions need to be made about staffing resources required—the kind of staff (OTRs, COTAs, aides, secretaries, etc.) and the number of staff. The kind of staff required will be determined by the services the program will offer and the skill level needed to perform the services. The number of staff needed can be determined by

Table 10-1
Examples of Program Goals and Objectives

Program:	Community Re-entry Skills Program
Goal:	To expand services to head injury in- and outpatients by including community re-entry skill activities in their treatment regimen.
Objective:	75% of the patients treated in the community re-entry skills program will demonstrate improved ability to handle themselves in a community setting.
Program:	Pediatric Mental Health Occupational Therapy Evaluation
Goal:	To provide developmental screening for children hospitalized on the mental health unit.
Objective:	85% of the patients referred to the pediatric mental health unit will receive developmental screenings.
Program:	Injured Worker Program
Goal:	To increase OT's referral sources.
Objective:	Increase the number of contracts within the area for the injured worker program by two within the next year.

plotting out the hours needed to carry out patient treatment activities, documentation, meetings, and preparation/follow-up. It may be helpful to lay out a mock work schedule based on projected volumes. Time should be allowed for lunch and break times as well.

Step 4—Financial Implications

The financial implications of a program include both the program's costs and revenues. At this point in the program development process, the program is clearly outlined and it is time to allocate costs to the resources which will be used and to estimate what probable revenues or income may be.

Costs

Costs basically fall into two categories: initial start-up costs and operating expenses. Start-up costs would include all supplies and equipment (both capital and non-capital) which will need to be purchased and available for use when the program begins. Renovation costs to the space to be used should be considered. If it will be necessary to hire staff or use current staff time to prepare for the program before it opens, these hours and their costs should also be included, as well as any training costs. Marketing and promotions costs also need to be included. Operating expenses are those costs accrued by the program after it begins. Ongoing supply, equipment, and staffing costs are included. Generally, operating expenses are estimated for the first year of operation.

Revenue

At this stage the planners must determine whether the program will be a revenue-producing service or whether its costs will be absorbed by the department or organization. Some programs that may not involve direct patient treatment or for which reimbursement is not available may not be revenue producing. If the program will produce revenue, then fees for services provided must be established. Different fees may be established for different services such as individual treatment, group treatment, evaluations, splints, etc., or fees already established by the department may be used. The *Uniform Terminology* document may be a helpful resource to guide decisions about categories of services to charge. If new fees are to be established the following information should be considered:

- Actual costs involved in providing the service
- What reimbursers currently pay for services and policies regarding payment
- What other providers charge for similar services

Consultation with the financial manager of the institution is recommended to determine whether fees charged cover all expenses, a portion of expenses, or all expenses plus a profit. In most cases the fee needs to be high enough to cover costs and allow for a margin of profit, yet low enough to be within the range of charges allowed by reimbursers and/or charged by other providers in the area.

After the fees are established, the total revenue is estimated by multiplying the volume estimated for each service times the fee charged for each service. Adding together the revenue produced for each service will provide the planners with the total revenue projected for the new program.

Comparison of Costs and Revenues

A direct comparison of cost and revenue will reveal that the program makes money, loses money, or breaks even (revenues cover costs). Depending upon the philosophy of the organization in which the program resides, one or several of the above may be preferable. Program planners would be wise to be aware that this "bottom line" figure will often have a strong influence on the program's viability and acceptance within the organization. If the bottom line demonstrates a loss, the program may need to be reconsidered by re-evaluating volume projections, costs, and fees for service.

Step 5—Implementation Plan

The last step of the program development process is the design of a plan for implementing the program. All facets of the program have now been described. The planners know where the program will take place, what supplies and equipment are needed, and what staffing is required. They have wrestled with how the program will look and what different activities will occur within the program. Now the planners must sort out the separate tasks that must be accomplished to bring the program into being. As the tasks are identified they should be plotted along a timeline with target dates for completion noted.

In the implementation plan, consideration should be given to the tasks that need to be carried out in the following areas.

Space Preparation

The physical space where the program will be housed may need to be acquired, renovated, or arranged. If the program is to be housed in the current space, some equipment may need to be moved and/or other changes made. Plans and target dates for moving will need to be made.

Supplies and Equipment

Necessary items will need to be ordered in time to allow for delivery, installation, and stocking before the start of the new program.

Activity Preparation

The policies, procedures, and protocols for the activities that will be part of the program need to be developed. Although these may change after the program is underway, the staff involved in the program need to think out some basic procedures ahead of time in order to direct their actions in the beginning of the program.

Staff Preparation

Personnel to staff the new program will need to be recruited and hired. Job descriptions also need to be developed. Current and newly hired staff may need additional training if new skills are needed for the proposed program. Orientation to program goals, objectives, and protocols for all staff will be required before the program opens.

Promotion

Plans for marketing the program to clients and referral sources are essential for the success of the program. How are people to be notified about this new service? Is a brochure needed? Newspaper coverage? Individual contact with referral sources? The chapter on marketing in this book further discusses this topic.

Evaluation

A plan for evaluating the effectiveness and success of the program should be formulated as part of the implementation plan. Criteria for determining the success of the program and a procedure for collecting the necessary data need to be built into the plan. Two kinds of criteria should be considered—process evaluation criteria and outcome evaluation criteria. Process evaluation criteria will focus on the way the program has been conducted. For example, all evaluations were completed within two treatment sessions. Outcome evaluation criteria will focus on the results of the program. They measure the program's outcomes. For example, 75% of patients treated in the work hardening program will return to gainful employment by the completion of the program. The program's objectives, if they have been specifically and measurably written, should form the basis of the program's outcome evaluation.

Writing the Program Proposal

Producing a written document that presents and summarizes all the thinking and planning of the program developers is the culmination of the process. The hard work is finished. The planners now take their information and organize it for others to review. The written program proposal provides a record of the planning process and should answer all basic questions about the program's purpose, content, and benefits. A suggested program proposal outline is presented in Table 10-2.

Most of the information to be included in the written proposal has already been generated during the program development process. However, program benefits and risks and uncertainties have not been specifically addressed.

As the planners near the end of the program development process, they should have a clear idea of the program's benefits and potential risks. The financial benefits have been clearly outlined under financial implications. They can be briefly summarized and restated here along with other quantitative benefits such as productivity, change in market share, or effectiveness. Qualitative benefits that may be more difficult to quantify should not be overlooked. The effect of the new program on the organization's image, influence, and quality of care may be significant. Risks and uncertainties associated with rapidly changing conditions or current problems might influence the viability of the program and should be noted. Changing government or reimburser policies, pending legislation, and risk associated with being able to recruit staff are possible examples.

Table 10-2
Outline for a Written Program Proposal

I. **Purpose and Justification**
   A. Purpose of program
   B. Problem the program addresses
   C. Assessment of need

II. **Description**
   A. Program description
   B. Implementation plan

III. **Analysis of Costs and Benefits**
   A. Financial implications
   B. Program benefits
   C. Risks and uncertainties

IV. **Summary and Conclusions**

The Planning Process

Since the program development process is a sequential one and new information is being gathered and developed along the way, there are several points at which the planner may pause to re-evaluate whether the program is still worthwhile and whether to continue the process. For example, if the needs assessment demonstrates that the actual need for or utilization of the proposed program would be minimal, the planners may decide that further development of the program is unnecessary. Likewise, if during the program description step it becomes apparent that costs to set up the program are becoming excessive, the planners may choose to stop the process or scale down their original idea to make it less costly.

The steps in the process have been presented in a logical sequence. However, in actuality steps may overlap or information acquired in one step may require the planners to go back to a previous step. Planning is a continuous process and is never truly completed in the sense that new information may require the planners to revise previous plans.

Conclusion

The program development process allows the planners to think through their ideas in a logical and comprehensive manner. Facts are gathered to support ideas and conclusions. The process allows the planners to anticipate problems and minimize failure. A program that has been well planned has a greater chance of running smoothly and being successful. Good planning is the cornerstone to effective programming.

Questions

1. A program is:
    a. Any activity carried out in an OT department
    b. An activity that involves patient treatment only
    c. A specially designed service aimed toward a specific goal
    d. All of the above

2. Ideas for new programs come from:
    a. The marketing department
    b. Patients and families
    c. Other health care providers
    d. All of the above

3. Which of the following statements does not describe the program development process?
    a. The process is composed of sequential steps
    b. Once started all the steps of the process must be completed
    c. The process allows the planners to anticipate possible problems
    d. The process requires the planners to support their ideas with factual data

4. Program development is the responsibility of:
    a. The department manager
    b. The senior supervising therapist
    c. The staff therapist
    d. All of the above

5. The step of the program development process in which the planners gather factual information to document the existence of the problem is called:
    a. The idea
    b. The needs assessment
    c. The program description
    d. The financial implications

6. When the planner is describing the program in Step 3, which of the following is not addressed?
    a. The program's benefits
    b. The outline of the program's activities
    c. The target population
    d. The program's usage of resources

7. The purpose of the needs assessment step is:
    a. To convince others of the need for your program
    b. To assess the needs of the patients targeted for your program
    c. To begin to market your program
    d. To factually support the extent of the problem your program will address

8. Which of the following factors should be considered when establishing fees?
    a. Costs involved in providing the service
    b. What others charge for the same or similar service
    c. What reimbursers will pay for the service
    d. All of the above

9. Which of the following is true about program goals and objectives?
    a. Goals and objectives are the same thing
    b. They should be consistent with the organization's direction and mission
    c. Once set, they should not be changed
    d. They are nice to have but are not an important aspect of the program development process

10. The statement "85% of the patients referred to the pediatric mental health unit will receive developmental screenings" is an example of which type of evaluation criteria?
    a. Process evaluation criteria
    b. Outcome evaluation criteria

Case Study 1

Shelley is an OT who works in a pediatric outpatient clinic treating children ages 4 to 14 with sensory integration dysfunction and mild to moderate developmental delays resulting in learning disabilities. Every summer for the past several years she has listened to the parents of her clients complain about the lack of available structured summer activities for their children. She has also noticed that the social skills and judgment of her clients are deficient and has struggled with how she could more effectively address these needs in her 1:1 therapy program. She decides that perhaps both of these needs could be addressed in a new program—a summer play camp offered in her outpatient clinic. Her target population would be children 6 to 11 years of age with developmental delays.

Shelley shares her idea with the OT manager who agrees that it has merit and asks her to develop a program proposal for the idea. As she begins thinking about her idea she defines an initial goal for the proposed program—to study the need for a structured group program which would improve social skills in the child with developmental delays and learning disabilities.

To verify whether or not a need exists for her program Shelley conducts a survey of the parents whose children she has treated within the past 3 years. Survey response is overwhelmingly positive. Parents would be very interested in a summer program. She also contacts several local schools for the learning disabled and interviews their directors. The directors also confirm the need for such a program and are able to give her estimates of the number of children who might be appropriate and interested.

Based on the information gathered, Shelley confirms the need for the program and now begins to work out the details of the program's description. She refines her goal to "provide a structured group experience for learning disabled children aimed at improving social skills." The specific objective of the program will be "to improve social skills as measured on a social skills indicator in 75% of the children participating in the program." She decides that her target population should include any learning disabled child in the community ages 6 to 11. She proposes that the program be conducted in the gymnasium and recreation space of a nearby church. With equipment available from the clinic and the church, further major equipment will not be needed, but some expendable supplies, such as media and cooking supplies, will be needed. Shelley draws up a sample program of activities for the summer camp and decides she will propose running one 4-week session. After consideration of the kind of activities that will be conducted and the number of possible campers, she decides that the program can be run with one OTR and an aide. Based on the information she received from her parent survey and interviews with school directors she estimates that 10 to 15 campers may be interested.

She now sits down with the department's manager and specifically outlines start-up costs and operating expenses. A fee for the camp session that will cover expenses plus make a small profit is set.

Together Shelley and the manager map out the implementation plan and develop a timeline for sequence in which tasks to get the program running need to be accomplished.

The information that has been developed is compiled into a written proposal and submitted for approval.

Case Study 2

Ann is the manager of the OT department in a 400-bed hospital in a medium-sized midwestern city. The hospital's board of trustees, responding to decreasing demands for inpatient services, has decided to expand the mission of the hospital to include outreach to nearby communities. The hospital's OT department has had a tradition of attracting and retaining a capable and stable workforce due to the variety of its programming and effectiveness of its management. However, fluctuating inpatient caseloads have lowered productivity.

As manager, Ann is aware of several smaller hospitals within a 70-mile radius that have been unable to recruit and retain OT staff. She sees an opportunity to support the mission of the hospital, make more efficient use of her staff's time, and assist hospitals in need of OT services. She proposes the development of a new program to provide contract OT services to area hospitals.

After discussing the proposed idea with her administrator, she proceeds to conduct a needs assessment by collecting data from area hospitals. She discovers three hospitals that have been unable to provide OT services for 5 of the past 9 months. The administrators estimate that their average caseload varies from two to five patients per day in each hospital. The administrators contacted appear interested in exploring a way to provide more consistent service.

Ann proceeds to outline the program description as follows:

- Goal statement—To improve the availability of OT services in local medical institutions by providing outreach OT contract services.
- Objective—Increase department revenues by 15% and staff productivity by 20%.
- Target population—Patients referred to OT in area hospitals.
- Setting—OT clinics in area hospitals.
- Program activities—Patient evaluation and treatment.
- Volume—Approximately 6 to 15 patients will be treated per day at three different sites. Amount of therapist time required to carry out this activity is estimated at 6 to 20 hours per day plus travel time.
- Resource utilization—Space, equipment, and supplies will be provided by the host hospitals. One to one and one half OTRs will be required to carry out the program.

Financial implications were next determined by comparing costs and projected revenues. Initial start-up costs were minimal, involving basically the time required to negotiate contracts with the three hospitals. Operating costs included the therapists' salaries, benefits, and travel costs to the three facilities. Revenues were projected based on an hourly fee established for contract services. Multiplying the hourly fee times the estimated number of therapist hours required yielded the total revenue the program would generate. Revenues exceeded costs and therefore the program was considered to be financially viable.

A brief implementation plan was outlined which focused on orienting and preparing staff for contract work and outlining policies and protocols.

Suggested Readings

American Occupational Therapy Association. (1994). Uniform terminology for occupational therapy (3rd ed.). *Am J Occup Ther, 48*(11), 1048-1059.

Anthony, R. N., & Herzlinger, R. E. (1975). *Programming: New programs in management control in nonprofit organizations.* Homewood, IL: Richard D. Irwin, Inc.

Budgen, C. M. (1987). Modeling a method for program development. *J Nurs Adm, 17,* 19-25.

Dignan, M. B., & Carr, P. A. (1987). *Program planning for health education and health promotion.* Philadelphia: Lea & Febiger.

Haw, M., Claus, E., Durbin-Lafferty, E., & Iverson, S. (1984). Improving nursing morale in a climate of cost containment. Part 2: Program planning. *J Nurs Adm, 11,* 10-15.

Kiritz, N. J., & Mundel, J. (1987). *Program planning & proposal writing introductory version.* Los Angeles: Grantsmanship Center.

Mayer, R. (1985). *Policy and program planning: A developmental perspective.* Englewood Cliffs, NJ: Prentice Hall, Inc.

McDonald, P. (1977). *Program development: Program and project planning and review.* Boise, ID: Health Policy Analysis and Accountability Network, Inc.

Persly, N., Slavin, W., & Albuny, S. (1988). Marketing rehabilitation programs. In *Marketing Everybody's Business Symposium Digest* (pp. 115-117). Chicago: American Marketing Association.

Scammahorn, G. (1985). Program planning. In J. Bair & M. Gray (Eds.), *The occupational therapy manager.* Rockville, MD: American Occupational Therapy Association.

Twain, D. (1983). *Creating change in social settings: Planned program development.* New York: Praeger Publisher.

Van de Ven, A. (1980a). Problem solving, planning, and innovation. Part I. Test of the program planning model. *Human Relations, 33,* 711-740.

Van de Ven, A. (1980b). Problem solving, planning, and innovation. Part II. Speculations for theory and practice. *Human Relations, 33,* 757-779.

Answer Key

1. c
2. d
3. b
4. d
5. b
6. a
7. d
8. d
9. b
10. a

CHAPTER 11

Designing Fieldwork Education Programs

Mary Farrell, MS, OTR/L

Definition and Purpose of Fieldwork Education

Fieldwork education is the time in an OT student's learning experience when the application of the academic coursework joins and clarifies theory and clinical practice. Fieldwork education is an on-site presence of an OT or OTA student in a health care or human service setting supervised by a fieldwork educator. This crucial aspect of OT education creates the opportunity for the student to develop insight into his or her understanding of him- or herself in a professional career, to implement the practical integration of academic knowledge and human responses to intervention, and to achieve competence in a challenging and competitive field.

Fieldwork education is integrated into the academic program at different intervals of the student's program. The AOTA *Essentials and Guidelines of an Accredited Educational Program for the Occupational Therapist* and *Essentials and Guidelines of an Approved Educational Program for the Occupational Therapy Assistant* require two levels of fieldwork experience as part of every curriculum. All students are required to complete a Level I fieldwork experience that is integrated into the academic program, and a Level II fieldwork experience that serves as the cornerstone of their professional entry-level education. This chapter will present fieldwork education as defined by the AOTA and outline the roles and responsibilities of the student, the clinical facility, and the school. Then, the issue of designing and evaluating the fieldwork education experience will be examined from the viewpoint of the student, clinical facility, and academic program.

Levels of Fieldwork Education

The AOTA identifies fieldwork education in two distinct levels. Level I is described by the AOTA as "experiences designed to enrich didactic coursework for the purpose of directed observation and participation in selected fieldwork settings." Level I fieldwork is customarily positioned in the academic curriculum after the student satisfactorily completes introductory courses in OT, biological sciences, and humanities. At this stage, the student has a cursory understanding of the field of OT and is prepared to pair this knowledge with field observation, beginning interview skills, and task analysis. Specific objectives for Level I fieldwork are collaboratively developed by the academic program and a fieldwork educator from the clinical site. While an OTR or COTA is typically the Level I supervisor, supervision may be provided by other professionals who are knowledgeable in the role of OT and the Level I fieldwork experience. The format of a Level I experience is set forth by the academic program, dependent on the position of the experience in the curriculum and the objectives. Frequently, Level I fieldwork is 1 to 2 weeks of on-site observation by the student to appreciate the flow of work, patient care, professional socialization, and administrative functions of a practitioner in a clinic. Level I fieldwork experience may also be integrated into coursework and follow a weekly schedule to enrich a particular didactic course content with very specific objectives.

Level II fieldwork is the in-depth clinical experience for students completing their academic requirements and is the final preparation for the certification examination and entry into the profession. In the *Guidelines for an Occupational Therapy Fieldwork Experience—Level II*, the Commission on Education states, "Level II fieldwork shall be required and designed to promote clinical reasoning and reflective practice, to transmit the values and beliefs that enable the application of ethics related to the profession, to communicate and model professionalism as a developmental process and a career responsibility, and to develop and expand a repertoire of OT assessments and treatment interventions related to human performance" (AOTA, 1992, 1993). OTA students are required to complete 12 weeks of Level II fieldwork; 6 months of supervised Level II fieldwork education is required for the OT student. Requirements for standards beyond the AOTA minimum may be established by the sponsoring academic program. The student is required to fulfill these requirements in order to be eligible to sit for the certification examination. Supervision for Level II fieldwork must be provided by an OTR or COTA with a minimum of 1 year's experience in OT practice. Fieldwork education may be any site that provides OT service. This broad definition includes a variety of delivery models, diagnostic consumer groups with various psychosocial and physical performance disabilities, and administrative or research operations. Level II fieldwork experience is the integration of didactic with practical education. In light of this, AOTA requires that all fieldwork experiences are completed within 24 months following the completion of the academic coursework for an OT student and within 18 months for an OTA student. The sponsoring academic program determines the eligibility of the student for the qualifying examination by its philosophy and mission. In some instances, the student receives the academic degree only after successful completion of the Level II fieldwork requirement. For other educational programs, the academic coursework completes the requirement for the academic degree and the fieldwork experience is required for the student's eligibility to sit for the certification examination.

Roles and Major Functions

Fieldwork education requires the collaboration of many individuals with the client as the core. The roles of the participants and their major functions are outlined here.

Client

The recipient of the service is the beneficiary of a well-planned and implemented OT fieldwork education program. The consumer is knowledgeable of the presence of the supervised student and, whenever practical, fully participates with the fieldwork supervisor and OT student in the treatment selection and goal-setting process.

Student

OT students are the core of the academic program and the key players in the fieldwork experience. The student experiences fieldwork education throughout the academic program. The intent and design of the curriculum determine the placement of each phase of fieldwork education based on the stated objectives of the experiences. Students go out on Level I fieldwork experiences after the successful completion of basic coursework. The selection of the Level I site is the result of a decision reached by the academic fieldwork coordinator based on the philosophy of the academic program, the student needs, objectives for the associated course, and its sequence in the curriculum. This decision making early in the academic program establishes a professional and collaborative relationship with the academic fieldwork coordinator and sets the stage for more intense decisions for Level II fieldwork placement and career decisions. Students examine their learning style, personal strengths, support systems, financial state, ability to encounter adversity, and acceptance of change in the quest for the Level I placement. The student submits a request for placement based on the outcome of collaboration with the academic fieldwork coordinator. A placement is made based on the request and the availability of an appropriate site.

In Level I clinical education, the specific course will determine the student function and responsibilities. The first clinical experience may be observational and the objectives may be to document the student's observances in the clinic such as to interpret the site OT service objectives, identify the client population and their response to OT services and identify the frame of reference employed by the practitioners and the relationship of the health care personnel to one another. In later Level I fieldwork course objectives, the student may have assignments reflective of the specific coursework such as observational evaluations of psychosocial and physical dysfunctions in the client population, treatment plans, and resources after the client's discharge from OT services.

The student selection of Level II fieldwork sites is based on factors of availability of the site to the sponsoring academic program, conditions of the terms of agreement between the academic institution and the facility, the philosophy of the organization relative to the student needs, the experience of the supervising therapist(s), and practical particulars such as geographic location, student financial state, availability of transportation, and family support. These important elements must be addressed before the site selection is reviewed by the academic fieldwork coordinator for acting on the request and final site placement for the student.

The student fieldwork experience at Level II is the transition period between the role of student and professional. The student is required to examine the assets he or she brings to the fieldwork site. The student should be able to convey what he or she knows, determine when to ask questions, and exhibit how new learning is integrated into the known body of knowledge. The student must arrive at the Level II fieldwork site with a sound conceptual basis of OT and be able to communicate this for any diagnostic group or service base.

The success of the Level II fieldwork experience for the student is dependent largely on the student. Each successful student brings self-known strengths and needs for growth, and the basic quest for learning, personal attributes of flexibility, and adaptability (Herzberg, 1994). Additionally, valued characteristics of being open to new learning opportunities and the sincere belief that teamwork is shared wisdom create a successful experience for the student and the fieldwork educator. These characteristics traverse the provinces of clinical settings, diagnostic populations served, supervisor teaching styles, and geography. Professional behavior that the students need to exhibit and refine include accountability, respect, and accommodation for differences in others, nonjudgmental approach to all clients, and appreciation for cultural differences.

The OT or OTA student assumes responsibility for the clinical placement as soon as the assignment is established. The student contacts the site and introduces him- or herself to the fieldwork supervisor. If the student supervisor is different from the facility fieldwork coordinator, the student may address questions to the student supervisor. If an interview is required before the fieldwork education experience is planned, the student calls to arrange a convenient time for the facility-based interview. The purpose of the interview is usually to acquaint the student with the facility and the staff members. In the interview process, the supervisors determine the student's learning style, clinical interests, and professional manner. The student sees the facility physical plant, observes the OT staff interactions, observes the client population, and may be able to discern the teaching style of the student supervisor. The student provides the clinical site with information about who to contact in the event of an emergency and medical insurance coverage documentation. Either the student or the academic program provides the facility with proof of professional liability coverage for the student effective during the fieldwork experience. If the facility requires specific health information beyond the general health physical exam data, the student is responsible for providing this to the facility before the start of the affiliation.

The student must advise the fieldwork educator of any special learning needs he or she has prior to starting the clinical affiliation. This information is provided by the student and may be discussed with the academic faculty if the student has authorized a release of information for the academic program. Level II fieldwork objectives are a result of the collaboration between the academic program and the clinical facility. They largely represent the goal of entry-level performance by the student before the allotted completion time. Additionally, the clinical site may require that the student perform tasks or learning experiences related to the affiliation but not required by the academic program. These may include fabrication of an adaptive device for the department so the student demonstrates skill, knowledge, and resourcefulness or presentation of a case study or inservice to rehabilitation personnel to fulfill similar objectives. Specific objectives for successful completion of Level II fieldwork education experience are clearly identified by the AOTA *Fieldwork Evaluation Form for Occupational Therapy Students* and the *Fieldwork Evaluation Form for Occupational Therapy Assistant Students*. Criterion scores are identified for the aggregate evaluation. Some academic programs have higher standards for passing scores or have identified letter grades for each experience based on the total score summary. While on the Level II clinical fieldwork education experience, the student adheres to the performance standards of the clinical facility just as other staff members do. During this educational experience, the student is also learning how to be a good supervisee and accept direction from the clinical educator to improve clinical performance. The student abides by the standards established in the principles of *Occupational Therapy Code of Ethics* as revised by the Representative Assembly of the AOTA and *Standards of Practice*.

Fieldwork Educator—Practice Setting

An OTR or COTA who is currently certified by the NBCOT and licensed as required by the individual state and has at least 1 year experience in a practice setting, may serve in the capacity of fieldwork educator. Common titles for fieldwork educator roles include clinical educator, clinical fieldwork coordinator or clinical fieldwork supervisor, or simply fieldwork coordinator or supervisor. The role of the fieldwork educator may include functions of coordination of clinical education for the facility and/or direct supervision of fieldwork students. The coordinator will establish the clinical education plan and specific objectives in accordance with the facility philosophy and mission, the departmental requirements, and other policies relative to student presence. Coordinators of clinical education establish education program schedules, mete out supervisory assignments, and develop education and professional development plans for OT student supervisory responsibilities. This responsibility also includes establishing student program policies and procedures, assessment of risk for the facility, ensuring the quality of care for the client with student care, maintaining client care coverage according to departmental standards, and ensuring timely and accurate completion of the student evaluation tool. Since the student will contact the fieldwork educator as the student supervisor, the coordinator arranges the acquaintance interview and makes the student assignment as appropriate. During this interview, the fieldwork educator may ask the student about his or her learning style. It is at this time that the student may reveal specific needs for learning. If the student has signed an authorization for the academic program to release information about the student, the clinical educator may discuss the student with the academic faculty members. Otherwise, the student works with the fieldwork educator to map out a plan for a successful fieldwork experience.

Facility and departmental orientation and student education are directed by the fieldwork educator. The fieldwork coordinator is the facility liaison with the academic fieldwork coordinator for the student fieldwork experience. It is the responsibility of the fieldwork coordinator to contact the academic fieldwork coordinator in the event of difficult student behaviors or activities out of the ordinary of student performance.

In order to keep current with fieldwork education practices, the fieldwork educator is well served by maintaining membership in the AOTA Education Special Interest Section and communicating with other fieldwork educators in regional and national consortia directed in clinical education.

It is important that the hosting institution values education and demonstrates support for the fieldwork educator. The support takes many forms:

- Provision of resources for student education, especially for development of clinical and supervisory skills
- Allowance for student-supervisor interaction and acknowledgment of the non-revenue producing time
- Allowance for time to develop a facility-specific quality fieldwork program
- Stipend or salary recognition for this additional responsibility
- Time and expense for development and sustained relationships with other fieldwork educators
- Support of membership in professional organizations
- Recognition within the institution of this program and the efforts of everyone involved

Academic Fieldwork Coordinator

The academic OT program is represented by one or more academic fieldwork coordinators. This position serves as the liaison between the facility and the academic program for the purpose of on-site clinical education for the OT or OTA student. The academic fieldwork coordinator is the student advocate for successful completion of fieldwork education.

In order to assign students to fieldwork education sites, the academic fieldwork coordinator must be familiar with requirements for clinical fieldwork, AOTA objectives, the philosophy and mission of the academic institution and OT program, fieldwork site characteristics, student strengths and weaknesses, challenges and preferences, and regional cultural practices of fieldwork placements.

The academic fieldwork coordinator is ideally a clinician with a working knowledge of academic issues and student concerns. Specific tasks of the academic fieldwork coordinator encompass the following responsibilities—establish fieldwork sites through determining eligibility as a clinical education site; negotiate terms of agreement between the academic institution and the clinical facility; and assist in establishing the facility's goals and objectives for each level of student experience.

The student is the focus of the academic program and a key player in the fieldwork education environment. The academic fieldwork coordinator knows the academic curriculum and the appropriate sites for Level I and Level II fieldwork for student assignment. This knowledge of fieldwork sites is acquired by the academic fieldwork coordinator through the synthesis of information from the Fieldwork Data Form, communication with the facility fieldwork educators, and on-site visits. After the student has completed a clinical affiliation at this site, the academic fieldwork coordinator has additional information from the Student Evaluation of Fieldwork Experience (SEFWE) and student reports. Most academic programs conduct annual evaluations of the entire academic program and seek feedback from the fieldwork sites that identifies the program strengths, weaknesses, and opportunities for growth. This information is shared with the occupational faculty by the academic fieldwork coordinator as the clinician's perspective of the OT program.

As the student advocate, the academic fieldwork coordinator initiates the clinical contact for student fieldwork, prepares the student for the fieldwork experience, and creates and sustains communication with the clinical site for the benefit of the student while at the center. When occasional difficulties arise between the student and the fieldwork educator, the academic fieldwork coordinator is the facilitator and mediator between the principals for a favorable outcome. If the outcome necessitates withdrawal of the student from the clinical site, the academic fieldwork coordinator counsels the student in the cause of the withdrawal, seeking the student's ownership of part of the problem and coaching the student in appropriate behavior in future placements. The student has the responsibility to advise the next affiliation center of any potential difficulties or specific behavioral objectives that the student must address on this clinical affiliation. The fieldwork student's personal and educational information is protected by the Family Educational Rights and Privacy Act of 1974 (Buckley Amendment). The academic faculty member only shares student information when the student has signed a written consent identifying areas where information can be shared for specific purposes.

Cancellation of fieldwork placements is the bane of the academic fieldwork coordinator. Sites cancel on occasion when there is no alternative to suitable student placement due to staffing changes or other circumstances beyond the control of the facility clinical coordinator. Students cancel when severe circumstances prevent their attendance at the assigned clinical placement. It is the responsibility of the academic fieldwork coordinator to search for an appropriate replacement at the soonest opportunity.

Academic fieldwork coordinators maintain communication with other academic programs about trends and solutions to common fieldwork problems. With the abundance of academic programs, quality fieldwork placements are difficult to secure and maintain. Academic programs are working cooperatively to serve the needs of the students and the fieldwork sites.

Designing the Fieldwork Program

Serving as a fieldwork educator and sharing with students our affirmation for the profession is a primary way to contribute to the profession of OT (Cohn & Crist, 1995). In order to become a fieldwork site for clinical education of OT or OTA students, the practitioner may use the AOTA's Commission on Education issue *Guidelines for Occupational Therapy Fieldwork—Level I* and *Guidelines for an Occupational Therapy Fieldwork Experience—Level II* to provide direction in developing a fieldwork education program. Consider the commitment of having students for Level I as separate from Level II, and the diverse responsibilities between the role of the professional OT and OTA student before deciding which aspects of fieldwork education suit the institution best.

Clinical Fieldwork Site Responsibilities

The design of the fieldwork education program is unique to each facility. The fieldwork coordinator must answer the self-study questions: What are this facility's objectives? What is our belief of health care? What is our belief of education? How does OT integrate into this institution? Will administration support an OT fieldwork education program? The fieldwork education proposal for clinical sites starts by collecting data about the institution and the OT services. The clinical facility sponsoring an OT fieldwork placement should have current accreditation by the appropriate credentialing agency or meet standards established by the academic institution/program. The administrators and staff of the institution should understand the principles and philosophy of OT education and accept the responsibility of the implications of implementing this program. The organization must support the development and continuing process of student education with personnel, materials, and continued education for the fieldwork educators. Will there be adequate staff coverage to support a student program?

There is considerable time and energy devoted to creating the philosophy and mission of the fieldwork education program that must be allotted before the student objectives are prepared. Are there facility-based student behavioral objectives that are in congruence with the AOTA objectives and those of the academic program?

Will the department provide assistance to the student to secure housing, parking, and orientation to the area and professional organizations? Is there access to computers, word processors, libraries, Medline, e-mail, photocopiers, or other information mechanisms?

As clients are the core of any health care or human service, are there sufficient opportunities for student education within the current structure of service delivery? Is client care at this facility conducive to learning experiences? Must the student submit affidavits of criminal clearance or child abuse clearance?

Is there support among other professionals? Do members of the referral base appreciate and understand the role of students in the health care network? Are they approachable and willing to understand? Will these members allow their referral clients be treated by a student under supervision of an experienced OT practitioner?

Are other members of the service delivery team accepting of students? Do they have student programs that will be in alignment with the OT fieldwork program? Are there general education programs accessible to OT students such as continuing medical education, grand rounds, case conferences, and inservices? Is continuing education credit provided to the student for participation in these programs?

Is there interest among OT staff to support a fieldwork education program? Do staff members understand that a program is successful by the efforts of all members? Are there eligible staff members who are eager to accept students for Level I or Level II fieldwork experiences? Are there other academic programs interested in the facility as a fieldwork education site? Who will decide the rotation or selection of academic programs that may have students attend this facility? What compromises must staff members make to achieve a successful fieldwork education program?

Facility and departmental administrators concern themselves with the effect that student education will have on the client population and the productivity of paid staff members. Clients benefit from the delivery of service by an interested and dedicated professional-in-training. Students are very deliberate in their client performance evaluations and treatment plans and devote substantial energy to the correct method of care. They query the supervisor for any detail and justify their choice of evaluation tool, method, and treatment with current theoretical base and techniques. It would give evidence that each client receives added value when he or she is provided treatment by a well-supervised student.

A cost-benefit study of Level II fieldwork education was conducted and reported in 1987 (Shalik). The results indicated that costs generated in the first few weeks of the 12-week placement were generally recovered by the sixth week, with benefits gradually increasing, then declining slightly through the end of the fieldwork. Intangible benefits must also be brought to the surface for the appreciation of administrators—as previously identified, the student can be a source of modest increase in the departmental revenue, all other variables remaining constant; the student may be considered as a potential employee and costly employee orientation may be shortened due to the student experience; and the student arrives with fresh ideas and current theory from the academic program, so new approaches to existing problems may be addressed by the innovative student perspective.

The national trend toward increasing OT programs graduating more students and the general reduction of clinical sites due to the effects of managed care create the need for a higher ratio of students to fieldwork educators. The model of one fieldwork educator to two or more students is increasing its appeal for the facilities and academic programs. Facilities value collaboration between or among the students as practice in professional teamwork. There are various successful models of this mentoring relationship in the health care professions (Crist, 1995; Hengel & Romeo, 1995; Jung, Martin, Graden, & Awrey, 1994; Ladyshewsky, 1993; Nolinske, 1995).

Does the physical plant provide support for a student program? Is there adequate space for a student to meet privately with the fieldwork supervisor, practice treatment techniques, write notes in a quiet space, or to confer with the academic fieldwork coordinator?

Once these basic elements have been reviewed, communication with the academic program may start in earnest. Concurrent with this communication is the formulation of the departmental philosophy for fieldwork education, position descriptions and responsibilities for fieldwork coordinator, fieldwork educator and additional responsibilities of support staff members, student behavioral objectives, schedule of student responsibilities, creation of the student handbook, policies and procedures related to education programs, grievance procedures, communication mechanisms, and other related tasks.

Writing a Statement of Philosophy for a Fieldwork Education Program

Each clinical facility needs to define itself in its own beliefs about health care, the role of OT, and the position that education of the OT or OTA student plays in it. While it seems like an immense undertaking, answering the questions about the role that the clinical facility plays in the community, the place that OT holds in the institution, and what goals the OT fieldwork education program will fulfill in the overall plan will provide a complete philosophical statement.

Mission Statement

This statement is more directed toward the global action of the statement of philosophy. It is a directed affirmation specifically created for the fieldwork student program in an individual OT department at a specific health care organization. The facility-specific fieldwork education performance objectives will be extracted from elements of the mission statement. For example, if an element of the mission statement includes the intent that students completing fieldwork at a facility will be responsible professionals in their community, a performance objective will include community service activities.

Writing Performance Objectives

This is the basic level of expectations for the student education program. Similar to a client treatment program and goal statement, the performance objectives clearly define the desired outcome for the student in each phase of responsibility. The performance objectives identified by the AOTA in *Fieldwork Evaluation Form for Occupational Therapy Students* and *Fieldwork Evaluation Form for Occupational Therapy Assistant Students* are thorough and traverse the breadth of OT practice. Specific student goals may be added to these or individual statements to the AOTA forms to make them unique to the facility. It is wise for the writer to keep in mind that each objective must be written to answer these questions about the objective:

- Who is responsible?
- When should it be done?
- What is the outcome?
- In what manner should it be completed?

Like all well-written objectives, it needs to be realistic, understandable, measurable, behavioral, and achievable. Regular assessment of facility-based OT fieldwork objectives will determine their continued application to the student program.

Supervision

Each student arrives at the fieldwork site with unique learning needs specific to his or her level of education, background, cognitive developmental level, and expectations. Educational level, background, experience, and expectations can be discovered through interviews and the assembled data provided by the academic program. The cognitive developmental level is more difficult to discern yet equally important in the learning process. In collaboration with the student, the fieldwork educator must determine the most effective teaching-learning mechanism for this student experience. Personal qualities of organization, abstract thinking, problem solving, flexibility, and self-confidence are difficult to measure yet are hallmarks of a professional. The fieldwork educator is challenged to provide direction and supervision to the OT or OTA student that builds on the student's knowledge and integrates learning with these higher level functions. Open collaboration and a sincere desire to learn by both the educator and the student will establish this learning environment.

Academic Program Responsibilities

The academic program will send the facility a copy of a letter of agreement outlining the responsibilities of each partner in the agreement, the extent or declaration of freedom from liability, the rights and obligations of each, and the termination of the agreement. A facility may have specific requirements which must be included in the agreement which will require the careful review of the organization's legal counsel before signatures are completed or student scheduling may begin. A signed copy of the written agreement (contract) is maintained by each organization.

The academic program sets forth policies and procedures to provide a successful experience for the student in the fieldwork environment. Before the agreement is signed, the clinical facility receives a copy of the academic program curriculum; a statement of the academic institution's statement of philosophy, mission, and core objectives; the academic OT program's statement of philosophy, mission, and core objectives; and request for placement which may stimulate a current time frame in which to initiate the program. Furthermore, the academic program has policies and procedures to ensure communication between the facility and the academic program relative to the generic educational plan and the specific student education experience. The academic fieldwork coordinator shares the facility information with students for placement requests and advises the students of the strengths of each facility for the particular placement.

A site visit is planned prior to the student attendance whenever possible. The academic fieldwork coordinator maintains contact with the fieldwork coordinator or supervisor during the student experience on an intermittent basis to determine a general progression of student performance.

Encountering Student Difficulties

There are circumstances when the best plans do not work out for a variety of reasons. If the student encounters difficulties while on clinical affiliation, the academic fieldwork coordinator must be notified as soon as possible regarding the issue. If the facility coordinator feels that the issue is easily solvable, the academic fieldwork coordinator is simply apprised of progress toward goals. If the situation becomes more serious and warrants intervention by the academic fieldwork coordinator, a site visit or telephone conference is held to facilitate a favorable outcome.

Under all circumstances, the fieldwork educator has the responsibility to determine the student's competencies in entry-level practice. If difficulties confronted exceed any capacity to resolve, it is the obligation of the fieldwork educator to fail the student in order to maintain high standards of practice and utilize this experience for an opportunity for growth for the student (Ilott, 1995). The academic fieldwork coordinator in collaboration with the academic program is the arbitrator of fieldwork placement issues.

Student Evaluation

Through ongoing supervision with the fieldwork educator, the student is kept aware of progress toward achieving the stated objectives. Halfway through the fieldwork experience a formal evaluation is conducted measuring the student performance against outcome objectives. The final outcome instruments, *Fieldwork Evaluation Form for Occupational Therapy Assistant Students* and *Fieldwork Evaluation Form for Occupational Therapy Students* are used with modification to assess the student's progress toward the goal of entry-level performance. The same evaluation tools are used at the conclusion of the student's fieldwork experience, this time with numerical values for scoring. The AOTA has established criterion scores for each subcategory of the evaluation. Some academic programs have higher standards for passing scores or have identified letter grades for each experience based on the total score summary. The student must achieve the recommended minimum passing score in each area to pass the fieldwork experience.

The facility may have additional standards by which the student is evaluated for which entry-level is defined at that institution.

Fieldwork Education Program Evaluation

During the student experience, the responses of the key players to the student presence are invaluable in ongoing assessment of the education program. Was there sufficient preparation for the student presence here? Were the important individuals included in the planning? Was there an oversight in the communication network? Was the academic program sufficiently involved? Did every participant feel valued?

The student's feedback directly relates to the fieldwork educator and the program at that time. Through the SEFWE, the fieldwork educator has specific feedback about supervision, client contact, the adequacy of resources, and the experience as a whole in response to the student needs. The clinical facility retains a copy of the SEFWE for its records, and the original is returned to the school for continued assessment of the facility by the academic program. The original is housed in the fieldwork files for future fieldwork students' review for selection for clinical placement.

The fieldwork coordinator at the clinical site has many issues for consideration. Was there an interruption in client service due to the presence of the student? How was the department enriched by the student? When can the department accept another student? Has the collaborative model of student supervision been explored? Were student objectives achieved? If not, why not? Could the student have had a broader experience? Could the department have been more open to the student experience? Next time, will the student be eligible to observe a surgical procedure? Attend a health clinic? Represent the department at a wellness screening?

Program Evaluation—Academic

The academic program evaluates its process and outcome with various methods. The most direct assessment is the outcome of the national certification examination by the students from the academic program. Additionally, feedback from clinical sites about individual and aggregate student performance, student competencies against stated objectives, the attentiveness of the academic faculty to the clinical facility, and direct student input from academic and fieldwork courses provide the academic program with valuable information about its program. Comments and feedback from clinical educators about the students and the supporting curriculum is sought and valued by academic programs.

Conclusion

Fieldwork education is the student's vital link between the classroom and a professional career in OT. Practitioners are educators of clients, families, and other health professionals. A primary role of the clinical practitioner is fieldwork educator for OT and OTA students. The fieldwork educator is a vital link from the present to the future of OT.

Questions

1. Fieldwork education is:
   a. Required for all students
   b. Required for only OT students
   c. The last step in becoming an OT practitioner
   d. Only provided in hospitals

2. A fieldwork educator may be:
   a. Any OT
   b. Any licensed OT
   c. Any licensed OT practitioner with 1 year of clinical experience
   d. Any person selected by the academic fieldwork coordinator

3. The OT or OTA student may:
   a. Complete fieldwork education wherever it is convenient
   b. Finish fieldwork education within 3 years of graduation
   c. Collaborate fieldwork education plans with the academic fieldwork coordinator

4. The fieldwork educator may be:
   a. A clinician
   b. A department administrator
   c. An OT practitioner
   d. All of the above

5. The *Fieldwork Evaluation Form for Occupational Therapy Assistant Students* and the *Fieldwork Evaluation Form for Occupational Therapy Students* may be used:
   a. As guidelines for progress
   b. Halfway through the affiliation with modified scoring
   c. As the primary evaluation for OT and OTA students
   d. All of the above

6. The fieldwork education program must be supported by the organization because:
   a. The administrator wants to know why revenue is down
   b. The referring physician wants to know why students are treating his or her patients
   c. Everyone who participates has a vested interest in the positive outcome of the student program
   d. It is just the way things are done

7. Supervision of fieldwork students is:
   a. Done by fieldwork educators
   b. Continuous
   c. Two-way communication
   d. All of the above

8. If the student is experiencing difficulty on the fieldwork experience, the fieldwork educator:
   a. Contacts the academic fieldwork coordinator
   b. Asks the student what issues are interfering with the fieldwork experience
   c. Discusses the situation with the fieldwork coordinator
   d. All of the above

9. The advantages of having fieldwork students are:
    a. Students stimulate higher awareness for client care by practitioners
    b. Students create enthusiasm for learning in a department
    c. The AOTA will look favorably on the department
    d. A and B and many other reasons

10. Fieldwork is:
    a. A primary responsibility of OT practitioners
    b. A significant part of a student's education
    c. Rewarding
    d. All of the above

Case Study 1

An OT fieldwork student has arrived on her first clinical affiliation at your subacute care facility. You have had several students from this particular academic program and are assured of the student's solid academic preparation. During the initial interview, you have determined that the student is goal-oriented and initiates activities of self-learning. The population base at this facility is neurological and orthopedic clients who were recently discharged from an acute care setting. Although the clients' medical status is stable, the acuity risk is high. The student presents her concerns about working with this population and expresses her anxiety to you. Since risk is an important issue with this diagnostic group, you work with this student to identify specific behaviors to ensure the clients' safety. The student's cognitive development level allows her to integrate new information into the existing knowledge base. She reviews texts about the specific diagnosis, refers to class notes, and studies the client's medical record for essential information particular to this person. She assesses and interviews the client using selected tools and seeks your confirmation of the data analysis. The student discusses her findings with other members of the health care team to discern appropriate discharge plans and needed community resources. The client, the student, and you decide which goals can be achieved through OT services.

The student has demonstrated self-knowledge, initiative, and adaptability, and has valued the team approach to client care. You have accurately assessed her need for guidance and direction and allowed her the level of independence appropriate to her abilities. Collaboration and mutual respect create the optimum learning environment.

Case Study 2

In a large urban rehabilitation hospital, an OT student is completing week 8 of the 12 weeks in her final fieldwork experience. There are students from many other academic programs, including OT and OTA students. The OT students are grouped in pairs or triads in this hospital according to work teams. Each small group works in a collaborative relationship and as part of the health care team for client care and problem solving. This student is grouped with another OT student from a local academic program and an OTA student from an established 2-year program. The group has worked together for 4 weeks on the neurological care unit and each member supports the others in patient care, mutual sharing of experiences, and problem solving. The senior student in her final month of clinical fieldwork serves as the coordinator and is learning skills of supervision of the OTA student. Under the direction of an OT supervisor, the student learns the complexities of supervision in client care, the satisfaction of collaboration, and the role of the professional in OT.

References

American Occupational Therapy Association. (1992). *Guidelines for occupational therapy fieldwork—Level I.*

American Occupational Therapy Association. (1993). *Guidelines for an occupational therapy fieldwork experience—Level II.*

Cohn, E. S., & Crist, P. (1995). Back to the future: New approaches to fieldwork education. *Am J Occup Ther, 49*, 103-106.

Crist, P. (1995, December 11). Making group-style fieldwork a success. *Advance for Occupational Therapy.*

Hengel, J. L., & Romeo, J. L. (1995). A group approach to mental health fieldwork. *Am J Occup Ther, 49*, 354-358.

Herzberg, G. L. (1994). The successful fieldwork student: Supervisor perceptions. *Am J Occup Ther, 48*, 817-823.

Ilott, I. (1995). To fail or not to fail? A course for fieldwork educators. *Am J Occup Ther, 49*, 250-255.

Jung, B., Martin, J., Graden, L., & Awrey, J. (1994). Fieldwork education: A shared supervision model. *Can J Occup Ther, 61*, 12-19.

Ladyshewsky, R. (1993). Clinical teaching and the 2:1 student-to-clinical instructor ratio. *J Phys Ther Educ, 7*, 31-35.

Nolinske, T. (1995). Multiple mentoring relationships facilitate learning during fieldwork. *Am J Occup Ther, 49*, 39-43.

Shalik, L. D. (1987). Cost-benefit analysis of level II fieldwork in occupational therapy. *Am J Occup Ther, 41*, 638-645.

Answer Key

1. a
2. c
3. c
4. d
5. d
6. c
7. d
8. d
9. d
10. d

APPENDIX A

American Occupational Therapy Association *Occupational Therapy Code of Ethics*

The American Occupational Therapy Association's *Code of Ethics* is a public statement of the values and principles used in promoting and maintaining high standards of behavior in occupational therapy. The American Occupational Therapy Association and its members are committed to furthering people's ability to function within their total environment. To this end, occupational therapy personnel provide services for individuals in any stage of health and illness to institutions, to other professionals and colleagues, to students, and to the general public.

The *Occupational Therapy Code of Ethics* is a set of principles that applies to occupational therapy personnel at all levels. The roles of practitioner (registered occupational therapist and certified occupational therapy assistant), educator, supervisor, administrator, consultant, fieldwork coordinator, faculty program director, researcher-scholar, entrepreneur, student, support staff member, and occupational therapy aide are assumed.

Any action that is in violation of the spirit and purpose of this Code shall be considered unethical. To ensure compliance with the Code, enforcement procedures are established and maintained by the Commission on Standards and Ethics. Acceptance of membership in the American Occupational Therapy Association commits members to adherence to the *Code of Ethics* and its enforcement procedures.

Principle 1. Occupational therapy personnel shall demonstrate a concern for the well-being of the recipients of their services (beneficence).

A. Occupational therapy personnel shall maintain services in an equitable manner for all individuals.

B. Occupational therapy personnel shall maintain relationships that do not exploit the recipient of services sexually, physically, emotionally, financially, socially, or in any other manner. Occupational therapy personnel shall avoid those relationships or activities that interfere with professional judgment and objectivity.

C. Occupational therapy personnel shall take all reasonable precautions to avoid harm to the recipient of services or to his or her property.

D. Occupational therapy personnel shall strive to ensure that fees are fair, reasonable, and commensurate with the service performed and are set with due regard for the service recipient's ability to pay.

Principle 2. Occupational therapy personnel shall respect the rights of the recipients of their services (autonomy, privacy, confidentiality).

A. Occupational therapy personnel shall collaborate with service recipients or their surrogate(s) in determining goals and priorities throughout the intervention process.
B. Occupational therapy personnel shall fully inform the service recipients of the nature, risks, and potential outcomes of any interventions.
C. Occupational therapy personnel shall obtain informed consent for subjects involved in research activities indicating they have been fully advised of the potential risks and outcomes.
D. Occupational therapy personnel shall respect the individual's right to refuse professional services or involvement in research or educational, practice, research or educational activities.
E. Occupational therapy personnel shall protect the confidential nature or information gained from educational, practice, research, and investigational activities.

Principle 3. Occupational therapy personnel shall achieve and continually maintain high standards of competence (duties).

A. Occupational therapy practitioners shall hold the appropriate national and state credentials for providing services.
B. Occupational therapy personnel shall use procedures that conform to the *Standards of Practice* of the American Occupational Therapy Association.
C. Occupational therapy personnel shall take responsibility for maintaining competence by participating in professional development and educational activities.
D. Occupational therapy personnel shall perform their duties on the basis of accurate and current information.
E. Occupational therapy practitioners shall protect service recipients by ensuring that duties assumed by or assigned to other occupational therapy personnel are commensurate with their qualifications and experience.
F. Occupational therapy practitioners shall provide appropriate supervision to individuals for whom the practitioners have supervisory responsibility.
G. Occupational therapists shall refer recipients to other service providers or consult with other service providers when additional knowledge and expertise are required.

Principle 4. Occupational therapy personnel shall comply with laws and Association policies guiding the profession of occupational therapy (justice).

A. Occupational therapy personnel shall understand and abide by applicable Association polices; local, state, and federal laws; and institutional rules.
B. Occupational therapy personnel shall inform employers, employees, and colleagues about those laws and Association policies that apply to the profession of occupational therapy.
C. Occupational therapy practitioners shall require those they supervise in occupational therapy related activities to adhere to the *Code of Ethics*.
D. Occupational therapy personnel shall accurately record all information related to professional activities.

Principle 5. Occupational therapy personnel shall provide accurate information about occupational therapy services (veracity).

A. Occupational therapy personnel shall accurately represent their qualifications, education, experience, training, and competence.
B. Occupational therapy personnel shall disclose any affiliations that may pose a conflict of interest.
C. Occupational therapy personnel shall refrain from using or participating in the use of any form of communication that contains false, fraudulent, deceptive, or unfair statements or claims.

Principle 6. Occupational therapy personnel shall treat colleagues and other professionals with fairness, discretion, and integrity (fidelity, veracity).

A. Occupational therapy personnel shall safeguard confidential information about colleagues and staff members.
B. Occupational therapy personnel shall accurately represent the qualifications, views, contributions, and findings of colleagues.
C. Occupational therapy personnel shall report any breaches of the *Code of Ethics* to the appropriate authority.

Prepared by the Commission on Standards and Ethics (SEC) (Ruth Hansen, PhD, OTR, FAOTA, Chairperson).
Approved by the Representative Assembly April 1977.
Revised 1979, 1988, 1994.
Adopted by the Representative Assembly, July 1994.
This document replaces the 1988 *Occupational Therapy Code of Ethics* (*Am J Occup Ther, 42*, 795-796), which was rescinded by the 1994 Representative Assembly.

Sources

American Occupational Therapy Association. (1994). Occupational therapy code of ethics. *Am J Occup Ther, 48*(11), 1037-1038.

APPENDIX B

American Occupational Therapy Association National Office Organization Chart

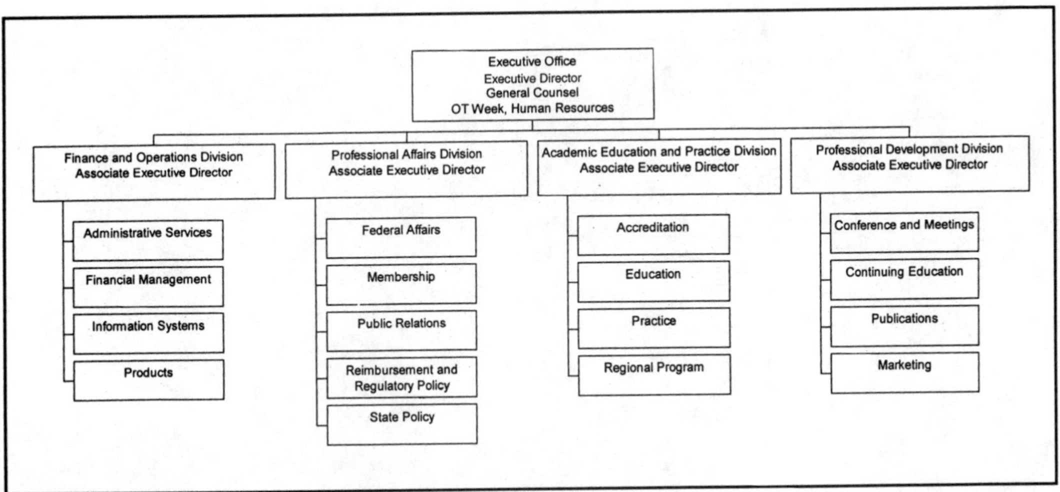

Courtesy of the American Occupational Therapy Association.

APPENDIX C

American Occupational Therapy Association Vision and Mission Statements

Vision Statement

AOTA advances occupational therapy as the preeminent profession in promoting the health, productivity, and quality of life of individuals and society through the therapeutic application of occupation.

June 1997

Revised: November 1997

Final: January 1998

Mission Statement

The mission of the American Occupational Therapy Association is to support a professional community of members and to develop and preserve the viability and relevance of the profession. The organization serves the interest of its members, represents the profession to the public, and promotes access to occupational therapy services.

June 1992

Courtesy of the American Occupational Therapy Association.

Index